Nutritional Meal Guide for Diabetes Reversal

A Comprehensive Approach to Naturally Reversing Diabetes.

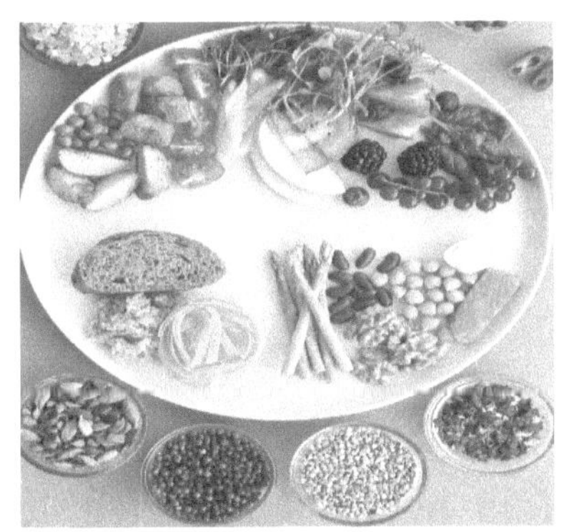

Efren R. Thomas

Copyright © (Efren R. Thomas), (2004)

No part of this book may be copied, distributed, or transmitted in any form or by any means, including photocopying, recording, or other electronic or mechanical methods, without the publisher's prior written permission, with the exception of brief quotations in critical reviews and certain other noncommercial uses permitted by copyright law.

Disclaimer:

The content in this book is intended for general informative purposes only. While every effort has been made to ensure that the content is accurate and complete, the author and publisher make no express or implied representations or warranties about the completeness, accuracy, reliability, suitability, or availability of the information, products, or services discussed.

The information contained in this book is not intended to diagnose, treat, cure, or prevent any illness. It is not an alternative to professional medical advice, diagnosis, or treatment.

Never reject or delay obtaining competent medical advice because of what you've read in this book. The author and publisher accept no responsibility for any errors or omissions in the content, nor for any actions taken based on the information provided.

Acknowledgements

Writing "Nutritional Meal Guide for Diabetes Reversal" has been a fantastic adventure, made possible by the encouragement, direction, and inspiration of so many lovely people. I'd want to express my heartfelt gratitude and appreciation to everyone who helped make this book possible.

First and foremost, I want to express my heartfelt gratitude to the distinguished authors whose breakthrough work has greatly influenced my understanding of diabetes treatment and nutrition. Dr. Richard K. Bernstein's "Dr. Bernstein's Diabetes Solution" has been a source of information and hope. His insights into diabetic care not only influenced my approach, but also pushed me to dive deeper into the field of nutritional therapy.

I am also grateful to Dr. Jason Fung, whose book "The Diabetes Code" provides essential insights into the science behind diabetes reversal through nutrition. His revolutionary approach to intermittent fasting and metabolic health has served as the foundation for the tactics presented in this book.

This book is more than just the result of my research and experiences; it is a monument to the collaborative efforts of people who inspired my journey.

Thank you for joining us on this journey and believing in the potential health transformation through the power of nutrition

With deepest gratitude,

Efren R. Thomas

Contents

Conclusion / Bonus

References.

INTRODUCTION

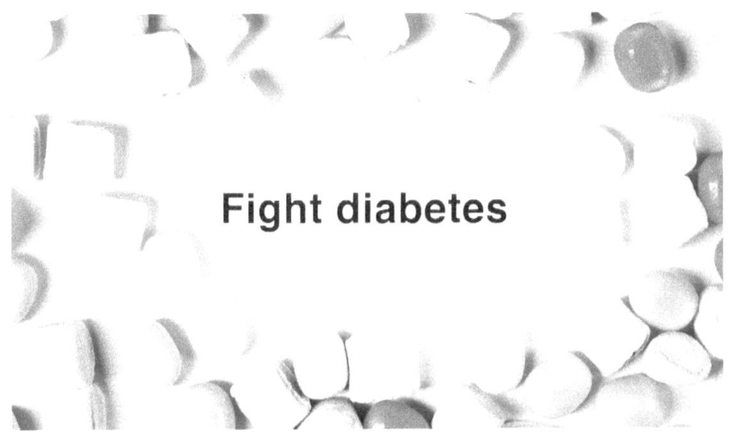

1. Welcome to Your Journey

Welcome to "**Nutritional Meal Plan for Diabetes Reversal: A Comprehensive Approach to Naturally Reversing Diabetes.**"

This book is more than just a collection of recipes and suggestions; it's a guide to living a healthier, more vibrant existence. Whether you've recently been diagnosed with diabetes or have been managing it for years, this book will provide you with the information and skills you need to take charge of your health.

Understanding Diabetes: An Overview

Let's start with your narrative. Imagine waking up every morning with a spring in your step, feeling energised and ready to face the world. If you've been dealing with diabetes's highs and lows, this may appear to be a distant dream. But it does not have to be. Understanding diabetes is the first step in regaining your health.

Diabetes is a chronic disorder that alters the way your body converts food into energy. When you consume, the majority of the food is broken down into sugar (glucose) and released into your bloodstream. When your blood sugar levels rise, your pancreas releases insulin, allowing the sugar to enter your cells and be used as energy. When you consume, the majority of the food is broken down into sugar (glucose) and released into your bloodstream. When your blood sugar levels rise, your pancreas releases insulin, allowing the sugar to enter your cells and be used as energy. For diabetics, this technique does not work properly.

There are two forms of diabetes. **Type 1 diabetes** is an autoimmune disease in which the body assaults insulin-producing cells in the pancreas. This form usually appears in childhood or adolescence, but it can occur at any age. Type 1 diabetes is treated with insulin for the rest of one's life.

Type 2 diabetes, which is more frequent, develops when your body becomes insulin resistant or produces insufficient insulin. It most commonly affects adults, but as obesity rates rise, an increasing number of children and teenagers are being diagnosed. Lifestyle factors, such as a poor diet and a lack of exercise, contribute significantly to the development of type 2 diabetes.

Diabetes care, regardless of type, includes regular blood sugar monitoring, medication, and lifestyle adjustments. While this may sound frightening, the good news is that with the appropriate treatment, type 2 diabetes may be managed and even reversed.

The Science Behind Diabetes Reversal

Reversing diabetes may sound too good to be true, but it is supported by science. Numerous studies have found that combining diet, exercise, and lifestyle changes can greatly improve blood sugar management and minimise or eliminate the need for medication in persons with type 2 diabetes.

Nutrition is central to reversing diabetes. What you eat has a significant impact on your blood sugar levels and general health. By eating the correct foods, you can control your blood sugar, reduce inflammation, and increase insulin sensitivity. This book will help you navigate these options by providing simple, effective recipes that are both delicious and healthful.

But how does a diabetes-reversing diet look like? It's high in complete, unprocessed foods. Think about colourful veggies, lean proteins, healthy fats, and entire grains. These foods not only help to regulate blood sugar but also give the nutrients your body requires to thrive.

One important principle is the balance of macronutrients (carbohydrates, proteins, and fats). Carbohydrates have the greatest impact on blood sugar, so choose them carefully. Choose complex carbohydrates such as whole grains and vegetables, which digest slowly and provide a consistent flow of glucose into the bloodstream. Protein and fats help to regulate blood sugar levels and keep you feeling full and satisfied.

Another important consideration is portion control. Eating the proper amount of food helps to reduce blood sugar rises and encourages weight loss, both of which are essential for controlling and treating diabetes. This book will show you how to properly portion your meals without feeling deprived.

Exercise is another effective diabetes reversal strategy. Regular physical activity lowers blood sugar, increases insulin sensitivity, and promotes weight loss. Whether it's a brisk stroll, a bike ride, or a yoga session, including movement into your daily routine can have a big impact.

How to Use This Book

This book is designed to be your companion on the journey to reversing diabetes. It's packed with practical advice, delicious recipes, and tips for creating a healthy lifestyle that works for you.

Chapter 1: The Basics of Diabetes provides a detailed explanation of what diabetes is, how it develops, and the impact it has on your body. Understanding the science behind the condition is crucial for managing it effectively.

Chapter 2: The Role of Nutrition in Diabetes explores how food affects blood sugar levels and the importance of a balanced diet. You'll learn about common myths and misconceptions and discover how to make smart food choices.

Chapter 3: Essential Nutrients for Diabetes Reversal delves into the different types of nutrients your body needs. You'll learn about the good and bad carbohydrates, the importance of proteins, and how to find the right balance of fats.

Chapter 4: Superfoods for Diabetes Management introduces you to the top foods to incorporate in your diet. Learn about the advantages of antioxidants and how to incorporate herbs and spices into your recipes.

Chapter 5: Creating a Diabetes-Reversing Meal Plan offers step-by-step instructions for setting realistic goals, balancing macronutrients, and regulating portions. You will also find information about meal scheduling and consistency.

Chapter 6: Grocery Shopping and Pantry Essentials explains how to create a diabetic-friendly kitchen.

Learn how to make grocery lists, read food labels, and stock up on nutritious staples.

Chapter 7: Meal Prep Strategies for Success provides practical advice on batch cooking, freezing meals, and creating quick and easy dishes. You'll also get tips on eating out and vacationing.

Chapter 8: Breakfast to Kickstart Your Day revolves around getting a good start in the morning. Discover energising smoothies, healthy breakfast bowls, and diabetes-friendly pancakes and waffles.

Chapter 9: Satisfying Lunches include ideas for robust salads, nutritious sandwiches, and grain bowls. These meals are intended to sustain you throughout the day.

Chapter 10: Nourishing Dinners focusses on meal options that are both nutritious and tasty. You'll find protein-rich main meals, flavourful vegetarian options, and comfort food makeovers.

Chapter 11: Healthy Snacks and Treats offers suggestions for nutritional snacks, guilt-free treats, and sensible desire solutions. Learn how to indulge in delicacies without jeopardising your health.

Chapter 12: Lifestyle and the Long Term Success emphasises the necessity of incorporating physical activity, managing stress, and tracking your progress. You'll find advice on remaining motivated and creating a support system.

Chapter 13: Appendices contains a dictionary of key concepts, extra resources and reading, and an index to assist you navigate the text. Throughout the book, you'll read inspiring accounts about people who successfully treated and reversed their diabetes via lifestyle modifications.

These stories demonstrate the strength of perseverance as well as the benefits of a good diet and regular exercise. This book does not promote quick cures or fad diets.

It is about making long-term improvements to your health. It's about taking control of your life and future. It is about recognising that you have the ability to modify your story. As you begin this journey, remember that progress, not perfection, is the aim.

There will be obstacles along the way, but each step puts you closer to a healthier, happier life. Use this book as a guide, motivational tool, and companion. Together, we can make the dream of reversing diabetes a reality. Welcome to your path towards a healthier future. Let's get started.

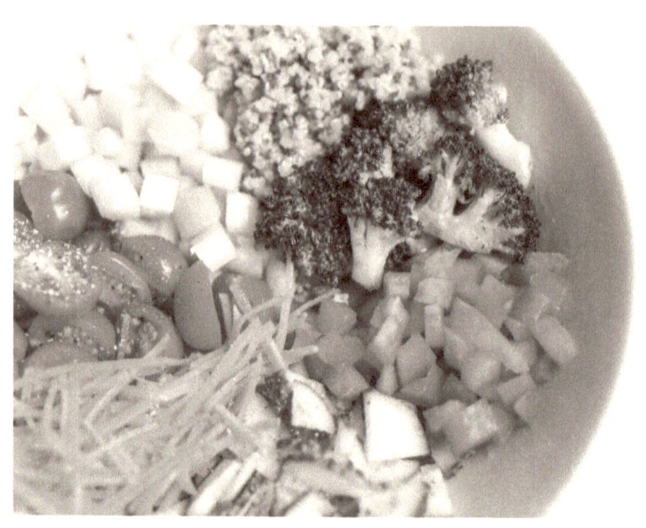

Part 1: Understanding the Basics of Diabetes

2. Diabetes Demystified:

Diabetes is a chronic health issue that affects how your body transforms food to energy. Normally, when you eat, your body breaks down the majority of the meal into sugar (glucose), which is then released into your bloodstream. When blood sugar levels rise, your pancreas secretes insulin. Insulin is a hormone that serves like a key, allowing blood sugar to enter your body's cells for usage as energy. In diabetes, this mechanism does not function properly. There are two basic forms of diabetes: Type 1 and Type 2. Additionally, gestational diabetes develops during pregnancy.

• **Type 1 diabetes** is an autoimmune disease in which the body assaults insulin-producing cells in the pancreas. As a result, the body produces little or no insulin. People with Type 1 diabetes must take insulin every day to live. This kind of diabetes is commonly diagnosed in children and young adults, but it can arise at any age.

• **Type 2 Diabetes:** This is the most common type of diabetes. Type 2 diabetes occurs when the body fails to appropriately use insulin. This is known as insulin resistance. Initially, the pancreas produces more insulin to compensate, but it cannot keep up over time, causing blood sugar levels to rise.

Type 2 diabetes is frequently associated with lifestyle factors and develops gradually. It is primarily diagnosed in adults, but it is becoming more common in children, teenagers, and young adults as obesity rates rise.

• **Hormonal Changes:** During pregnancy, the placenta generates substances that can make cells resistant to insulin.

• **Increased Demand for Insulin:** The demand for insulin rises as the pregnancy advances. If the pancreas does not create enough insulin to overcome resistance, blood sugar levels rise, resulting in gestational diabetes.

The Impact of Diabetes

Uncontrolled diabetes can cause a number of significant consequences. Over time, high blood sugar can damage blood vessels and nerves, resulting in difficulties like:

• **Heart Disease and Stroke:** Diabetes greatly raises the risk of cardiovascular disease.

• **Kidney Damage (Nephropathy):** Diabetes can harm the kidneys' filtering system, potentially resulting in kidney failure.

• **Eye Damage (Retinopathy):** High blood sugar levels can damage blood vessels in the retina, resulting in blindness if not treated.

• **Nerve Damage (Neuropathy):** Excess sugar can irritate the walls of the tiny blood vessels that supply your nerves, particularly in your legs. This can cause pain, tingling, or loss of sensation.

• **Foot Problems:** Poor blood flow and nerve damage in the feet increase the likelihood of different foot issues.

Managing Diabetes

Diabetes is effectively managed with a mix of lifestyle adjustments, monitoring, and medication. **Key strategies include:**

• **Healthy Eating:** A balanced diet high in whole foods, fibre, and low in processed sugars aids with blood sugar control.

• Regular exercise increases insulin sensitivity and benefits in weight management.

• **Blood Sugar Monitoring:** Regular monitoring allows you to keep track of your blood sugar levels and make educated changes to your food, exercise routine, and medications.

• **Medication:** Depending on the type and severity of diabetes, medicines or insulin therapy may be required to keep blood sugar levels under control.

Understanding diabetes and how it develops is critical for optimal management and prevention of complications. People with diabetes can have healthy and fulfilling lives with the right care and lifestyle changes.

3. The Role of Nutrition in Diabetes

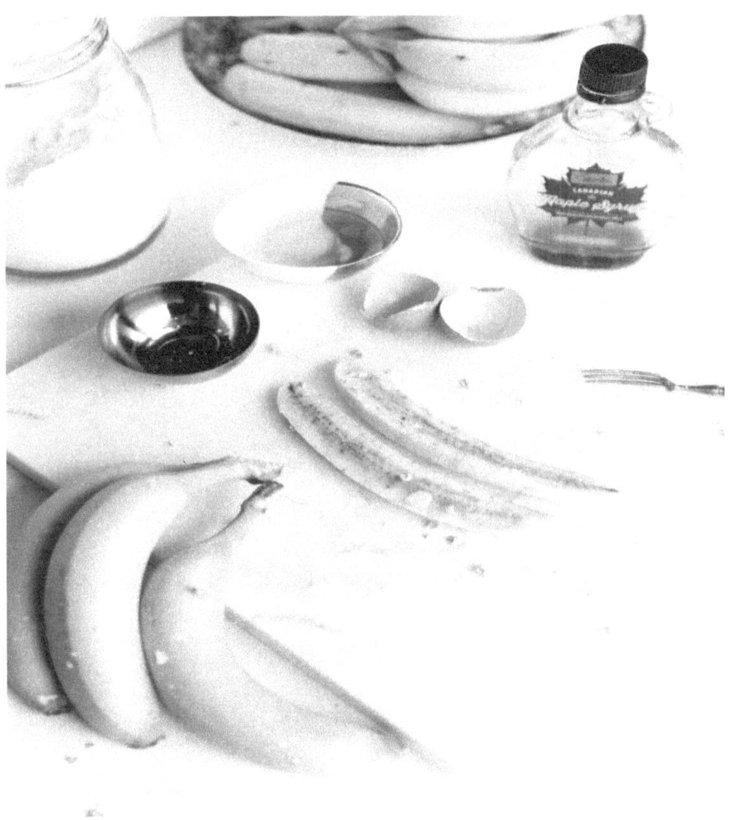

How Food Affects Blood Sugar:

Food plays a significant role in diabetes management, owing to its direct impact on blood sugar levels. When you eat, your body converts carbs into glucose, which enters the bloodstream. This increase in blood sugar causes the pancreas to secrete insulin, which aids cells in absorbing glucose for energy. Diabetes patients have compromised this mechanism, which results in high blood sugar levels.

- **carbohydrates:** Carbohydrates have the greatest impact on blood sugar. They can be found in foods including bread, pasta, grains, fruits, and desserts. Simple carbohydrates, such as sugar and processed wheat, induce a quick rise in blood sugar. Complex carbohydrates, such as whole grains and vegetables, are absorbed more slowly, resulting in a steady increase in blood sugar.

• **Proteins:** Although proteins do not have the same direct impact on blood sugar as carbohydrates, they are nonetheless important. Proteins aid in the repair and maintenance of human tissues and might indirectly affect blood sugar levels. Consuming protein alongside carbohydrates helps decrease the absorption of sugar into the bloodstream, reducing spikes.

• **Fats:** Fats have the least direct effect on blood sugar but are essential for general health. Avocados, almonds, and olive oil provide healthy fats, which can help reduce inflammation and enhance heart health. However, bad fats, particularly trans fats, can lead to insulin resistance and should be avoided.

The Importance of a Balanced Diet.

A healthy diet is necessary for everyone, but it is especially important for diabetics. Proper eating helps control blood sugar levels, maintains a healthy weight, and lowers the risk of diabetic complications.

• **Nutrient Variety:** A well-balanced diet consists of carbs, proteins, and fats. Each nutrient has a distinct purpose in supporting health. Carbohydrates give energy, proteins are necessary for development and repair, while lipids help cells function and produce hormones.

• **Portion control:** Understanding portion sizes is critical. Eating too many healthful meals can result in weight gain and elevated blood sugar levels. Using methods such as the plate approach, which fills half of the plate with non-starchy vegetables, a quarter with protein, and a quarter with carbohydrates, can help regulate portions more successfully.

• **Glycaemic Index:** Low-GI foods digest and absorb more slowly, resulting in a steady rise in blood sugar levels. Choosing low-GI meals such as whole grains, legumes, and non-starchy vegetables will help keep blood sugar levels constant.

• **Meal Timing:** Eating at regular intervals helps to keep blood sugar levels stable. Eating smaller, more frequent meals throughout the day can give a consistent amount of energy while keeping blood sugar levels stable.

Common Myths and Misconception

There are several myths and misconceptions concerning diabetes and nutrition, many of which can cause confusion and poor dietary decisions.

• **Myth:** All Carbohydrates are bad.

• **Reality:** Not all carbohydrates are made equal. Complex carbs, such as whole grains and vegetables, contain critical nutrients and should be included in a healthy diet. The idea is to consume high-quality carbohydrates in moderation.

• **Myth:** Diabetics cannot consume sugar. • **Reality:** Although sugary foods can raise blood sugar levels, diabetics can consume them in moderation. The emphasis should be on the overall quality of the diet rather than merely eliminating sugar completely.

Combining sweets with a balanced diet can assist to prevent blood sugar increases.

• There is no singular "diabetic" diet, contrary to popular belief. The greatest diabetes diet is one that incorporates a variety of nutrient-dense meals and is tailored to each person's specific needs and interests. The concepts of healthy nutrition are applicable to everyone, including diabetics.

• **Myth:** Consuming a lot of protein is best.
• **Reality:** While protein is essential, excessive protein intake can strain the kidneys, especially in diabetics. Balance is essential, as is getting enough carbs and good fats.

• **Myth:** Fat should be avoided.
The Truth: Not all fats are bad. Fish, almonds, and olive oil contain healthy fats that should be

consumed. The emphasis should be on avoiding unhealthy fats, such as trans and saturated fats, which can raise the risk of heart disease.

• **Myth:** Fruit is harmful to diabetics.
• **Fact:** While fruits contain natural sugars, they also give vital vitamins, minerals, and fibre. To avoid big blood sugar spikes, consider whole fruits over fruit juices and keep portion sizes under control.

Understanding how food affects blood sugar, the significance of a balanced diet, and refuting common misunderstandings can help people with diabetes make more educated decisions. A deliberate approach to eating is essential for successful diabetes treatment and general health.

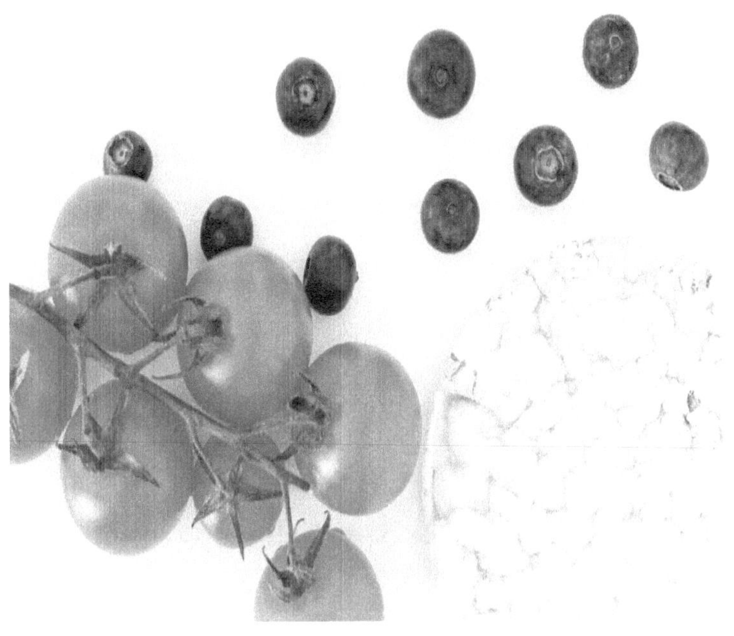

Part II: The Foundations of a Diabetes- Reversing Diet

4. Essential Nutrients for Diabetes Reversal

Carbohydrates: Good and Bad

Carbohydrates are important for diabetes management since they can have a significant impact on blood sugar levels. However, not all carbs are created equal.

• **Good Carbs:** These are complex carbohydrates found in foods such as whole grains, fruits, and vegetables. They digest slowly, which helps to keep our blood sugar stable and provides essential elements like fibre and vitamins.

• **Bad Carbs:** Think of these as simple sugars found in sugary drinks, sweets, and white bread. They cause rapid rises in blood sugar, which can be difficult to manage if you have diabetes. Consuming too many of them can result in weight gain and elevated blood sugar levels over time.

The idea is to focus on the beneficial carbohydrates. Choosing whole grains such as oats, brown rice, and whole wheat bread provides energy without causing abrupt blood sugar increases.

Proteins: Building Blocks of Health

Proteins are our bodies' superheroes, helping us build and repair tissues, maintain muscle strength, and even fight illness.

• **Protein-rich foods** include lean meats, fish, eggs, beans, almonds, and tofu. Combining protein and carbohydrates in your meals is beneficial since it lowers the rate at which your blood sugar rises after eating.

• **Benefits:** Protein makes you feel full and satisfied, which can keep you from overeating. It also helps your body mend and stay strong, which is especially important when controlling diabetes.

Just remember to choose lean proteins such as chicken without skin or beans over fatty meats. It's all about eating a variety of healthful foods to keep you feeling good.

Fats: Finding the Right Balance

Fats generally have a bad name, but they're actually quite beneficial to your health. They provide energy, protect your organs, and even assist your body absorb vitamins. However, just as with carbohydrates and proteins, there are good and bad fats.

• **Good Fats:** These are the unsaturated fats found in avocados, nuts, seeds, and olive oil. They can help keep your heart healthy and your blood sugar levels stable.

• **Bad Fats:** Avoid trans and saturated fats found in fried foods, pastries, and fatty meats. They can elevate bad cholesterol and increase your risk of heart disease.

To maintain balance, strive to eat meals with healthy fats most of the time. Use olive oil instead of butter, almonds instead of chips, and eat fish like salmon a few times a week to benefit your heart and blood sugar.

Understanding these critical nutrients—carbs, proteins, and fats—and how they influence your body can help you make better diabetes management decisions and feel better. It's all about figuring out what works for you and making little adjustments that hold over time.

5. Superfoods and Diabetes Management

Managing diabetes effectively entails selecting foods that can help control blood sugar levels and boost overall health. Here are some of the best superfoods, as well as antioxidant advantages and how to incorporate herbs and spices into your diet:

Include leafy greens, such as spinach, kale and Swiss chard, in your diet for high nutrition and low calorie intake. They're abundant in fibre and antioxidants, which can help protect against heart disease and regulate blood sugar levels.

• **Berries:** Blueberries, strawberries, and raspberries are high in antioxidants, vitamins, and fibre. They have a lower glycaemic index than many other fruits, resulting in a slower rise in blood sugar levels.

• **Fatty Fish:** Salmon, mackerel, and sardines are high in omega-3 fatty acids, which can lower inflammation and enhance cardiovascular health. They are also high in protein, which helps you feel full and pleased.

• **Nuts and Seeds:** Almonds, walnuts, chia seeds, and flaxseeds include healthful fats, protein, and fibre. They can help regulate blood sugar levels and lower the risk of heart disease.

• **Whole Grains:** Quinoa, barley, and oats are high in fibre and include essential elements such as magnesium and chromium. They digest more slowly than refined grains, helping to maintain steady blood sugar levels.

• **Yoghurt:** Select plain, low-fat yoghurt with no added sweeteners. Yoghurt contains probiotics (good bacteria), which may improve intestinal health and help control blood sugar levels.

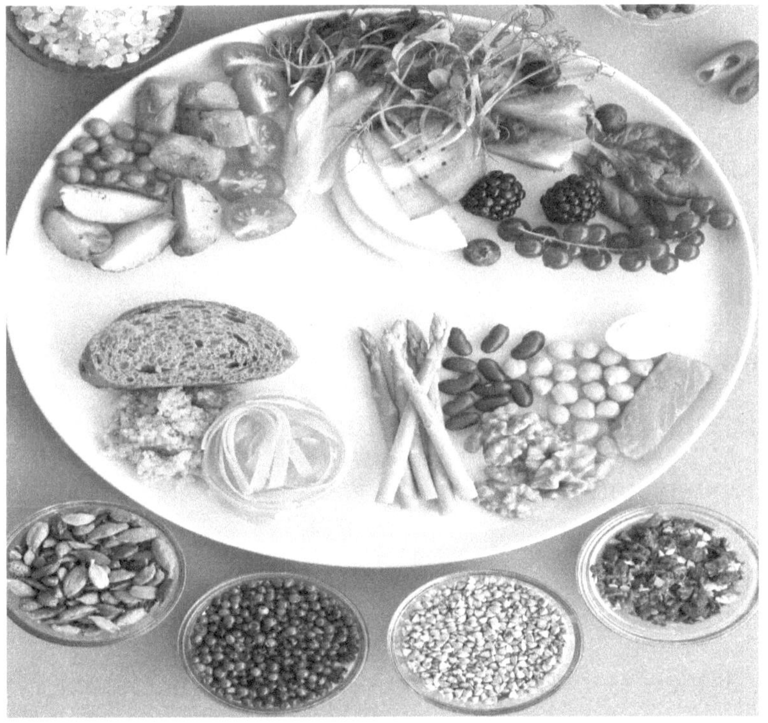

Antioxidants and their Benefits

Antioxidants are chemicals that protect our cells from free radical harm. Free radicals are unstable chemicals that damage cells and contribute to chronic diseases such as diabetes.

• Antioxidant-rich foods include berries, leafy greens, nuts, seeds, and colourful vegetables such as bell peppers and tomatoes.

• **Benefits:** Antioxidants reduce inflammation in the body, which is beneficial for diabetes management and reducing complications such as heart disease.

They also boost general immunological function and may increase insulin sensitivity.

Incorporating herbs and spices

Herbs and spices not only enhance the flavour of your food, but they also provide health benefits such as lowering blood sugar levels and inflammation.

• **Cinnamon:** This spice may increase insulin sensitivity and reduce blood sugar levels after meals. Sprinkle it over muesli, yoghurt or in smoothies.

• **Turmeric:** Turmeric is known for its anti-inflammatory effects, which can help reduce inflammation in the body. Add it to soups, golden milk, and curries.

• **Garlic:** Garlic can help decrease blood sugar and cholesterol levels. Use it in marinades, stir-fries, and roasted vegetables.

• **Ginger:** Studies have indicated that ginger improves insulin sensitivity and reduces inflammation. Use it fresh in tea, stir-fries, or on salads.

Incorporating these superfoods, antioxidants, and herbs/spices into your diet can help with blood sugar control, overall health, and lowering the risk of diabetic complications. It's all about creating delightful, nutrient-dense choices that will benefit both your health and your taste buds.

6. Developing a Diabetes-Reversing Meal

Setting Realistic Goals.

When creating diabetes reversal goals, be reasonable and specific. Begin with small, doable adjustments that can ultimately lead to a healthy lifestyle. How to Set Achievable Goals:

• **Set Specific Goals:** Rather than declaring "I want to eat healthier," try something more specific, such as "I will include a serving of vegetables in every meal." This gives you a clear, actionable step to do.

• **Make incremental changes:** Small steps might yield great results over time. For example, if you now consume sugary beverages on a daily basis, begin by reducing them to one per day, then every other day, and eventually replacing them with water or unsweetened drinks.

• **Monitor Your Progress:** Keep a food journal or use a mobile app to record what you eat and how you feel. This might help you stay accountable and track your progress.

• **Establish Timelines:** Give yourself a deadline to meet your objectives. This creates a sense of urgency and keeps you motivated.For example, strive to lose 5 pounds in a month or cut your daily sugar consumption in half over two weeks.

• **Celebrate Milestones:** Acknowledge and celebrate your accomplishments, no matter how minor. This positive reinforcement can drive you to maintain making healthy choices.

Balancing macronutrients

Balancing Macronutrients (carbohydrates, proteins, and fats) is critical for treating diabetes and sustaining good health.

- **carbohydrates:** Choose complex carbohydrates, such as whole grains, veggies, and legumes. These digest slowly, which helps to keep blood sugar levels constant. Avoid simple sweets and refined carbohydrates, as they might induce blood sugar rises.
- For example, instead of white rice, use brown rice or quinoa.

Proteins: Include lean proteins such chicken, fish, tofu, beans, and nuts. Proteins help you feel full and preserve muscle mass.

• For example, try grilled chicken breast with steamed broccoli and quinoa.

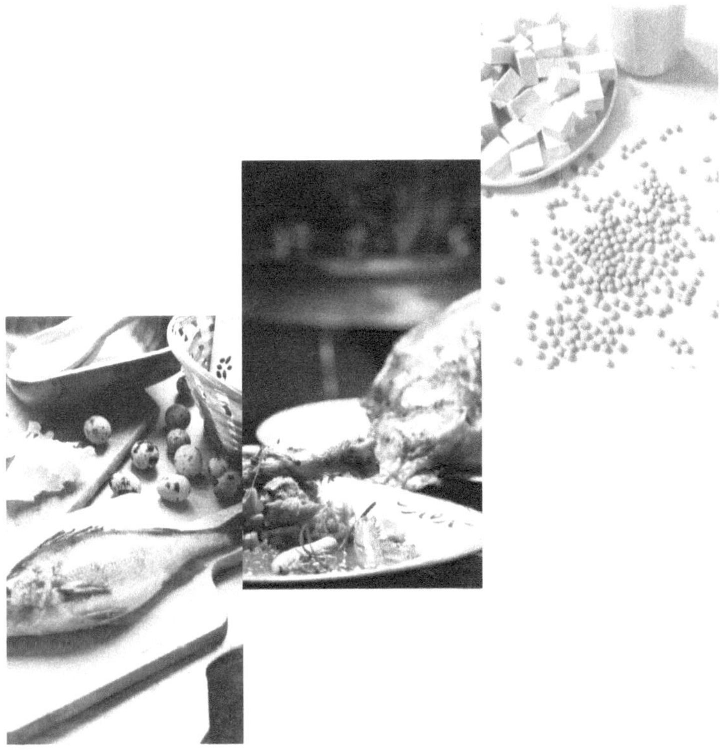

• **Fats:** Consume healthy fats like avocados, nuts, seeds, and olive oil. These fats promote heart health and help regulate blood sugar.

• For example, a salad treated with olive oil and
seeds.

Portion control and meal timing.

Portion control and meal timing are essential components of an effective diabetes-reversing diet. Here's how to get it correct:

• For better portion control, use smaller plates. Our brains frequently link a full plate with being full, so using a smaller dish can help you feel fuller with less food.

• Use measuring cups or a food scale to determine acceptable portion proportions. Over time, you'll get better at estimating portions without having to measure.

• **Mindful eating:** Slow down and savour every bite. Eating thoughtfully allows you to recognise when you are full and prevents overeating.

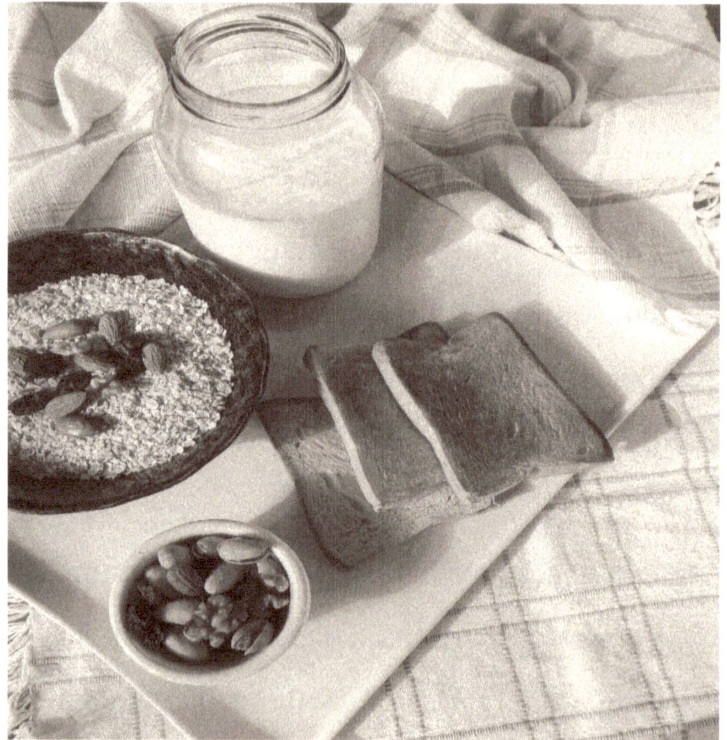

• **Meal Timing:** Eating at regular intervals promotes stable blood sugar levels. Aim for three main meals and two healthy snacks every day.

• **Don't Skip Meals:** Skipping meals might lead to overeating and fluctuating blood sugar levels. Always have a well-balanced breakfast to get your day started right.

• **Evening Eating:** Aim to finish your final meal a couple hours before bedtime. This allows your body to handle food more efficiently and maintains steady blood sugar levels overnight.

Setting realistic goals, balancing your macronutrients, and focussing on portion control and meal time will help you manage and potentially reverse diabetes. Making these adjustments gradually guarantees that they become long-term habits, which leads to improved health and well-being.

7. Grocery shopping and pantry essentials

Shopping Lists and Tips

Making a shopping list before going to the grocery store can help you save time, decrease stress, and adhere to your diabetes-friendly meal plan. Here are a few tips:

• **Plan Your Meals:** Before you go shopping, make a food plan for the week. Include a diverse range of proteins, veggies, complete grains, and healthy fats. This ensures you have all the necessary elements and prevents impulse purchases.

• **Organise Your List:** Combine comparable items on your list. For example, list all produce items, followed by dairy, proteins, and so on. This makes your purchasing experience more efficient.

• **Stick to the Perimeter:** The majority of fresh, healthy foods may be found along the store's perimeter. This includes fruits, vegetables, meat, and dairy items. Spend the most of your shopping time in these places.

• **Read labels.** Examine food labels for extra sugars, salt, and harmful fats. Choose things with fewer ingredients and avoid highly processed foods.

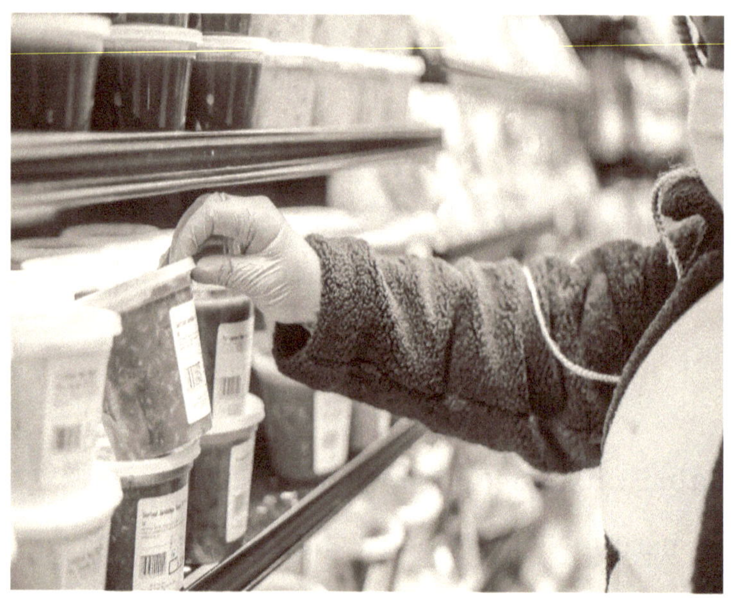

• **Buy in Bulk** (When Appropriate): Purchasing non-perishable foods in bulk, such as whole grains, beans, and nuts, can save money and minimise the number of shopping trips.

Stocking A Diabetes-Friendly Kitchen

A well-stocked kitchen makes it easier to cook nutritious meals and control diabetes. Here's how to keep your pantry, fridge, and freezer always stocked with nutritious options:

• **Pantry essentials**:

• **Whole grains** include brown rice, quinoa, muesli and whole wheat pasta.

• **Legumes** include canned or dry beans, lentils, and chickpeas.

• **Almonds,** walnuts, chia seeds, and flaxseeds are examples of **nuts and seeds.**

• Coconut oil, avocado oil, and olive oil are examples of **healthy oils.**

• **Spices and herbs** include cinnamon, turmeric, garlic powder, ginger, and dried herbs.

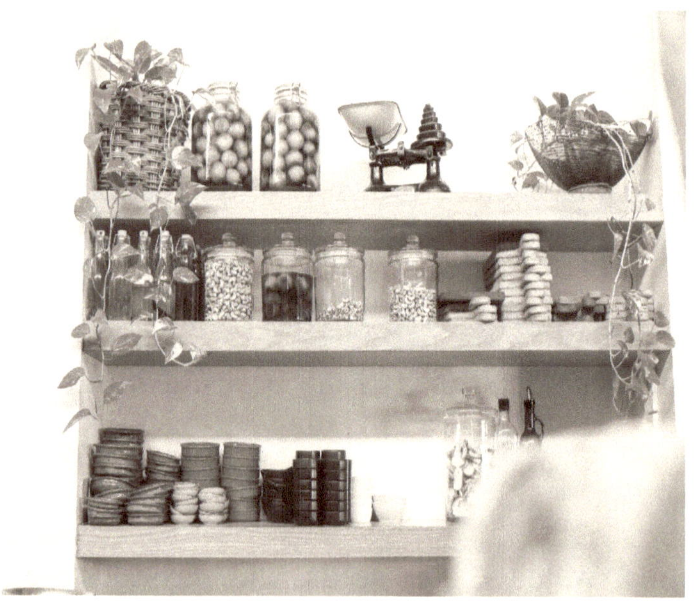

• **Refrigerator staples** include fresh vegetables like leafy greens, bell peppers, carrots, and cucumbers.

• **Fruits include** berries, apples, and oranges.

• **Lean proteins** include chicken breast, turkey, tofu, and low-fat dairy products.

• **Healthy snacks** include Greek yoghurt, hummus, and cut-up

• **Freezer essentials:**

• **Frozen vegetables** like broccoli, spinach, and mixed veggies.

• **Frozen fruits** include berries, mango, and peach slices.

• **Lean meats** include chicken breasts and fish fillets.

• **Prepared Meals:** Make soups, stews, or casseroles for quick meals

Reading and Understanding Food Labels

Understanding food labels is critical to making better choices. Here's how you decode them:

• **Serving Size:** Look for the serving size at the top of the label. All nutritional information is based on this amount, so if you consume more or less, you must modify the values accordingly.

• **Calories:** This indicates how much energy you get from a single dish. It is critical for controlling weight and total energy consumption.

• **Nutrients to Limit:** Check the levels of saturated fat, trans fat, cholesterol, and sodium. High doses can raise the risk of heart disease and high blood pressure.

• **Essential Nutrients:** Fibre, vitamins (such as A and C), calcium, and iron are all necessary for good health. Choose foods that contain higher levels of these nutrients.

• **Total Carbohydrates:** Includes sugars, complex carbohydrates, and fibre. Pay great attention to additional sugars. Aim for fiber-rich foods with few added sugars.

• **Ingredient List**: The ingredients are listed in order of quantity, highest to lowest. Look for complete foods first, and avoid goods with extensive lists of unfamiliar components.

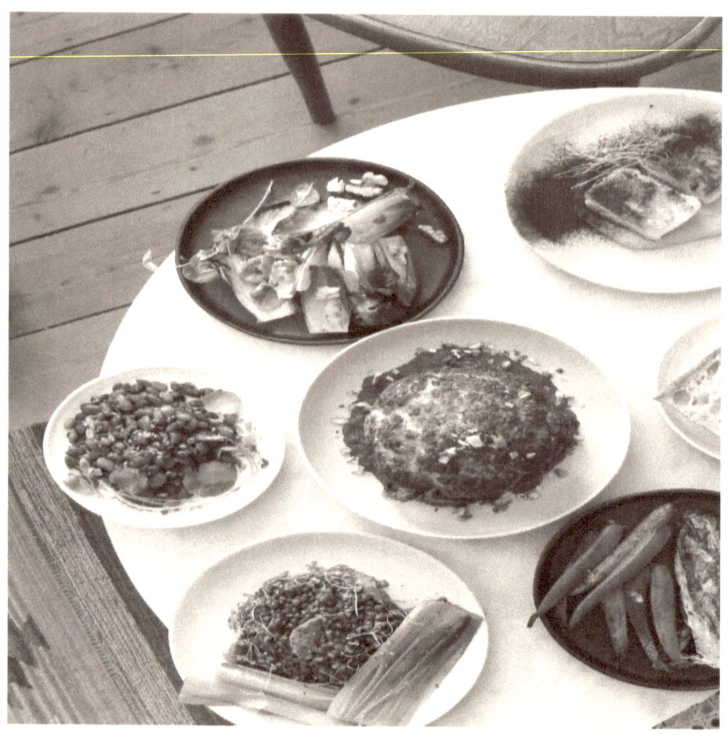

By following these shopping guidelines, stocking your kitchen with diabetes-friendly essentials, and understanding food labels, you can make healthier choices that help with diabetes control and general well-being.

8. Meal Preparation Strategies for Success

Batch Cooking and Freezing

Batch cooking and freezing meals can significantly improve diabetes management. It saves time, reduces stress, and ensures that you always have nutritious options on hand. Here's how to maximise the benefits of batch cooking:

• **Plan your recipes:** Choose a few diverse dishes that can be cooked in large batches. Soups, stews, casseroles, and chilli are great choices. They freeze nicely and are simply reheated.

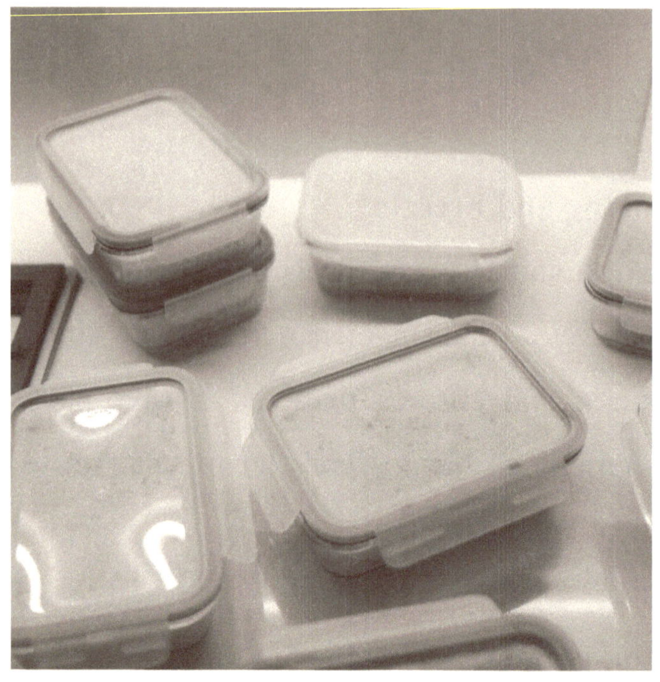

• **Cook in Bulk:** Set aside one day per week to prepare your meals. Cook huge quantities of each dish, divide them into individual containers, and mark them with the date.

- **Use Freezer-Friendly Containers**: Invest in high-quality, airtight containers designed for freezing. This helps to preserve the flavour and nutritional value of your food.

- **Freeze meals in single or family-sized amounts.** This allows you to defrost only what you need, saving waste and making meal preparation easier.

- **Rotate Your Stock:** Follow the "first in, first out" rule to ensure that older meals are used before newer ones. This prevents freezer burn and keeps your food fresh.

Quick and easy meal ideas

Sometimes you need healthful meals that can be prepared fast. Here are some suggestions for quick and easy diabetes-friendly meals:

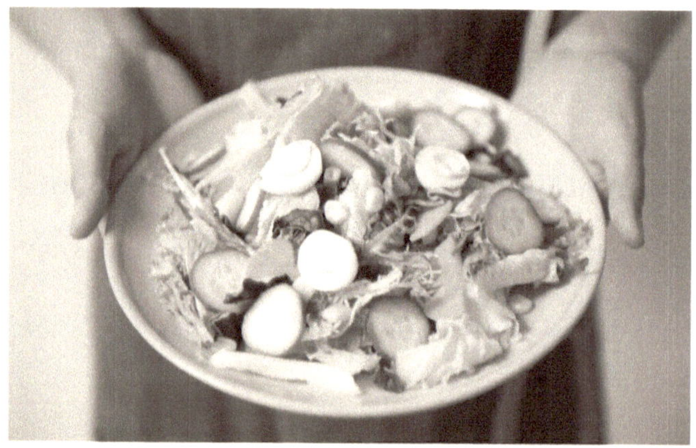

• **Salad bowls:** Combine a variety of greens with lean proteins such as grilled chicken, turkey, and tofu. Combine colourful vegetables, almonds, seeds, and a mild dressing.

• **Stir-Fries:** Stir-fries are quick and versatile. Sauté your favourite vegetables with lean protein (chicken, prawns or tofu) and a simple sauce of soy sauce, ginger and garlic.

• **Wraps and Sandwiches:** Fill whole-grain wraps or bread with lean proteins, vegetables, and a nutritious spread such as hummus or avocado.

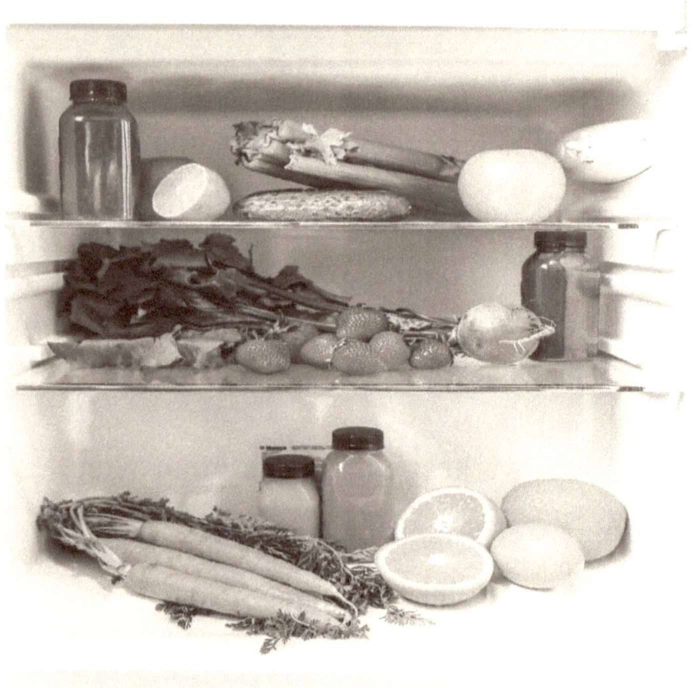

• **Smoothies:** Combine fruits, vegetables, and a protein source, such as Greek yoghurt or protein powder. Smoothies are ideal for breakfast or a quick snack.

• **Egg-based dishes:** Eggs are flexible and easy to cook. Make a vegetable-filled omelette or a frittata to portion out for the week.

Maintaining healthy eating habits while dining out or travelling can be difficult, but possible with little planning:

• **Plan Ahead:** Look up restaurant menus online before you go. Look for nutritious selections that fit within your meal plan, such as grilled meats, salads, and steaming vegetables.

• **Request Modifications:** Do not be afraid to ask for changes to your food. want dressing on the side, exchange fries for salad, or want grilled instead of fried items.

• **Keep an eye on portion sizes:** Restaurants frequently provide huge amounts. Before you begin eating, consider splitting a dish, requesting a half quantity, or packing half of your meal to take with you.

• **Choose Wisely at Buffets:** Begin with a salad to fill up on vegetables, then select lean proteins and avoid heavy sauces. Skip the bread and dessert sections.

• **Pack Healthy Snacks:** When travelling, bring along nutritious snacks such as almonds, fruit, whole-grain crackers, or yoghurt. This helps you avoid eating unhealthy foods when you're hungry.

• **Stay Hydrated:** Drink plenty of water, especially while travelling. Thirst can be mistaken for hunger, so staying hydrated might help you make smarter meal choices.

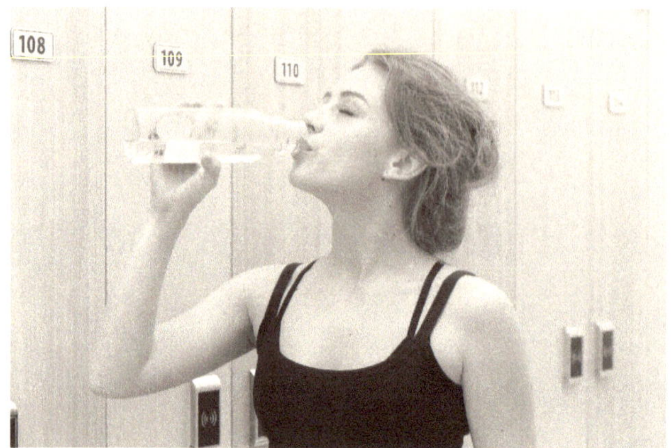

By using these meal prep ideas, you can integrate better eating into your daily routine, whether you're at home, out, or on the run.

Part IV: Delicious Recipes for Every Meal.

9. Breakfast to Start Your Day

Energising smoothies and shakes are a quick and nutritious way to start the day, especially for hectic mornings. Here's how to make tasty, diabetic-friendly smoothies:

• **Choose a base.** Begin with a nutritious liquid basis. Unsweetened almond milk, coconut water, and low-fat yoghurt are all viable options. These offer moisture and a creamy texture.

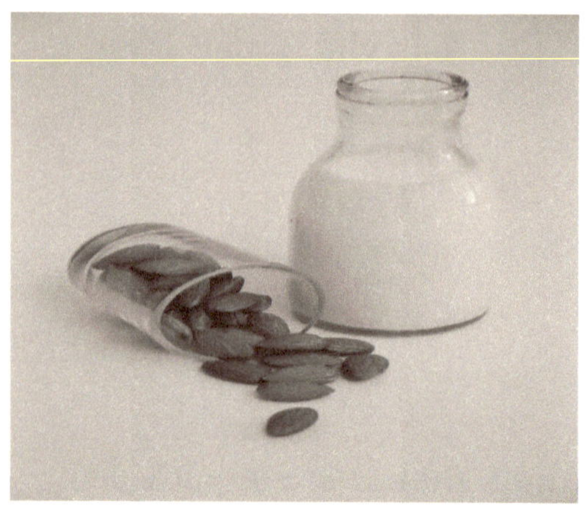

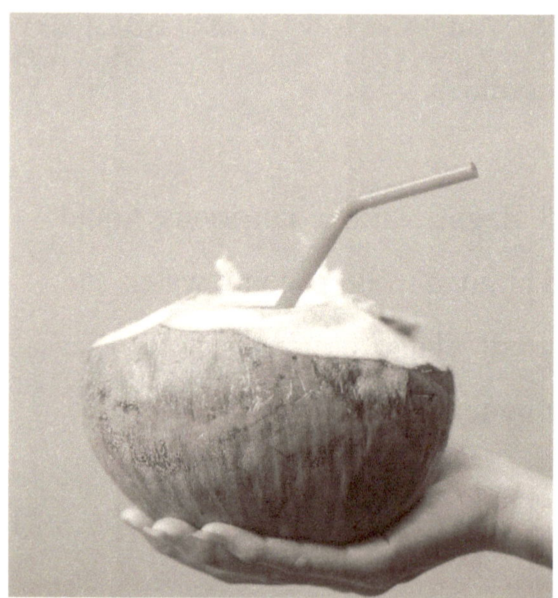

• Include a variety of fruits and vegetables for vitamins, minerals, and fibre. Berries, spinach, kale, and avocado all make excellent choices. These items are low in sugar but high in nutrition.

• **Include Protein:** Increase the protein level to keep you fuller for longer. Include Greek yoghurt, protein powder, or a handful of almonds and seeds. Protein helps to maintain blood sugar levels and offers prolonged energy.

• **Healthy Fats:** Include some healthy fats like chia seeds, flaxseeds, or a teaspoon of nut butter. These fats promote heart health and increase satiety.

• **Flavour Boosters:** Add natural flavourings such as cinnamon, vanilla extract, or fresh mint leaves to improve the taste.

- **Blend and Enjoy:** Place all ingredients in a blender and blend until smooth. Pour into a tumbler or a travel bottle for a healthful start to the day.

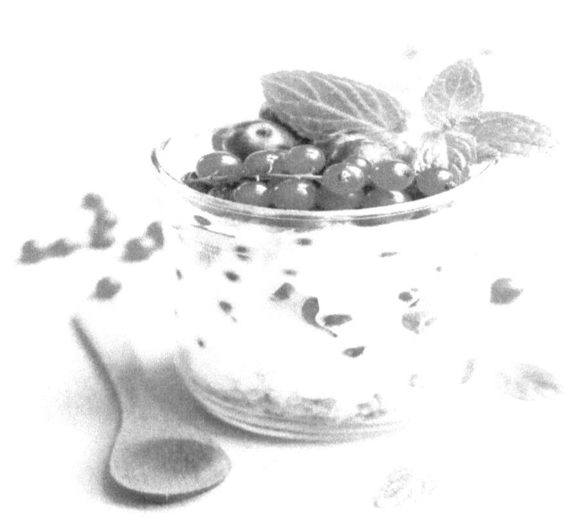

Nutritious Breakfast Bowls

Breakfast bowls are flexible and nutritious. They are simple to prepare and may be tailored to your preferences and nutritional requirements.

• **Base Ingredients:** Begin with a nutritious base, such as quinoa, muesli or Greek yoghurt. These give fibre, protein, and a sturdy base for your toppings.

• **Fresh Fruits:** Garnish your bowl with berries, apple slices, or bananas. They provide natural sweetness, vitamins, and antioxidants.

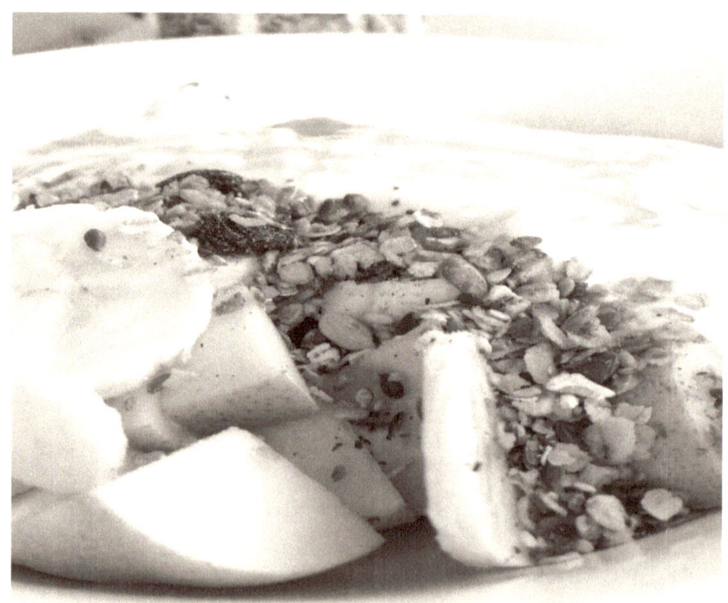

• Include healthy fats such as sliced avocado, almonds, and seeds. These substances add flavour and contain important fatty acids.

• **Protein Boost:** Try a poached egg, cottage cheese, or chia seeds. Protein helps to keep blood sugar levels stable and keeps you satisfied for longer.

• **Flavour and Texture:** Add some crunch and flavour with granola, coconut flakes, or a drizzle of honey. Choose low-sugar choices to keep it diabetic-friendly.

• **Combine and Serve:** Mix and match these ingredients to create a tasty and nutritious breakfast dish that energises

Diabetes-Friendly Pancakes & Waffles

Who does not adore pancakes and waffles? With a few modifications, you can enjoy these breakfast staples without raising your blood sugar.

• **Whole-Grain Flours:** Instead of refined white flour, use whole grains such as whole wheat, oat flour, or almond flour. These flours are rich in fibre and low in carbohydrates.

• **Natural sweeteners:** Instead of sugar, use mashed bananas, unsweetened applesauce, or a little amount of honey or maple syrup. These choices have a lower glycaemic impact.

• **Add Protein:** To increase the nutritional content, add protein powder, Greek yoghurt, or cottage cheese to the batter. This supplement helps you stay full and promotes muscle health.

• **Healthy Add-ins:** To increase fibre content and flavour, add nutrient-dense items such as chia seeds, flaxseeds, and berries.

• **Cook Smart:** Use a nonstick pan or a waffle iron to avoid the need for extra fat. If necessary, add a tiny amount of healthy oil, such as coconut or olive oil.

• **Top Wisely:** Choose nutritious toppings like fresh fruit, Greek yoghurt, or nuts. Avoid sweet syrups and whipped cream.

• **Serve and Enjoy:** Make a batch ahead of time and freeze individual servings for easy, healthy breakfasts all week.

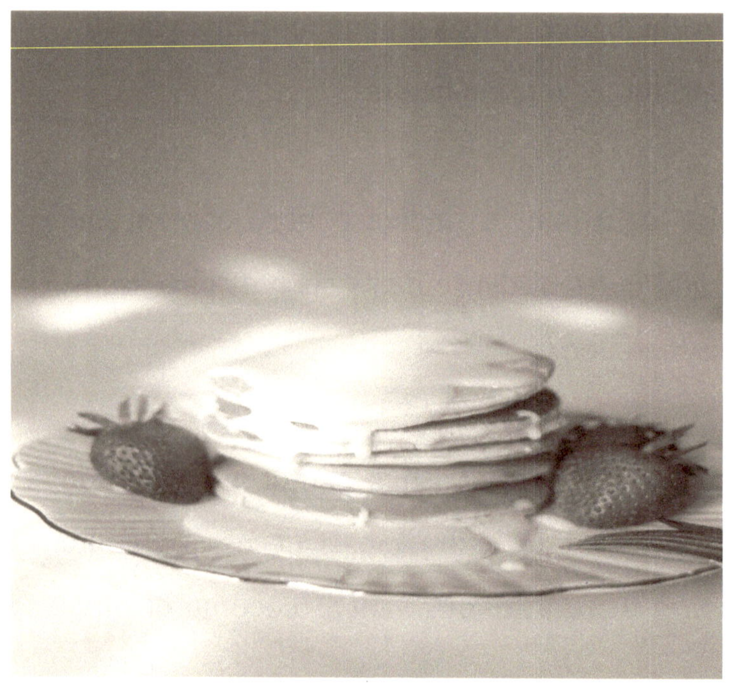

Starting your day with energising smoothies, nutritious breakfast bowls, or diabetes-friendly pancakes and waffles allows you to enjoy a range of delectable and healthy meals that will help you manage your diabetes and improve your overall health.

10. Satisfying lunches

Hearty salads and soups provide a variety of flavours and textures while maintaining stable blood sugar levels, making them a delightful and nutritious lunch option.

• **For hearty salads**, start with **base greens** like spinach, kale, rocket or mixed lettuce. These leafy greens are low in calories yet high in important nutrients such as vitamins A, C, and K.

• **Protein Punch:** Include a lean protein source to kccp you satiated and energised. Grilled chicken, turkey, tofu, and chickpeas are all wonderful options.

• **Colourful veggies**: Mix in a variety of veggies such as bell peppers, tomatoes, cucumbers, carrots, and beets. More colours equals more nutrients.

• **Healthy Fats**: Include healthy fats like avocado slices, almonds, and seeds. These enhance flavour while also aiding in the absorption of fat-soluble vitamins.

• Add a sprinkling of cheese, a handful of berries, or a boiled egg for more protein and flavour.

• **Light Dressing:** Prepare a light homemade dressing using olive oil, lemon juice, vinegar, and herbs. Avoid store-bought dressings, which are heavy in sugar and bad fats.

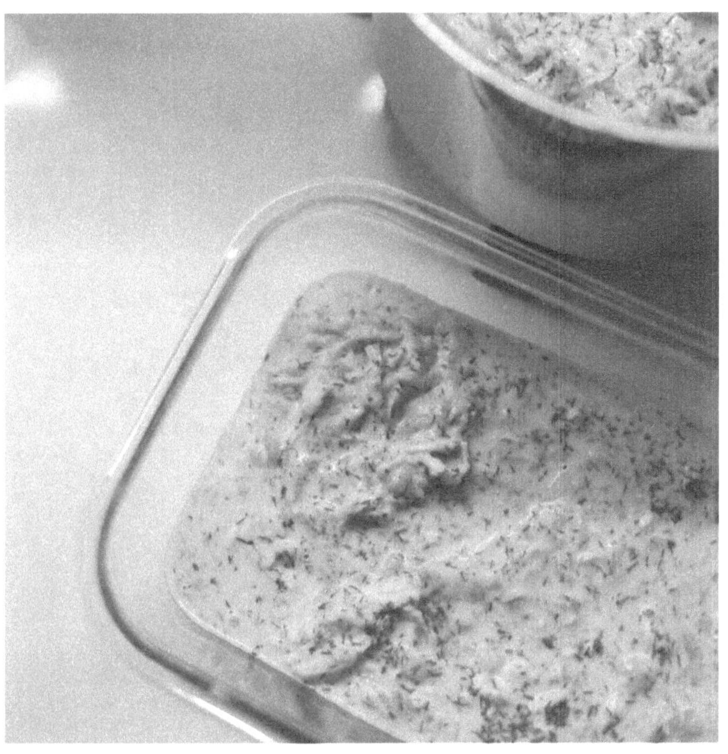

Nourishing soups

• **For nourishing soups**, start with a low-sodium base broth, such as chicken, beef, vegetable, or bone broth. This is the foundation of a healthy soup.

• **Lean Proteins**: Use shredded chicken, turkey, tofu, or beans. These components contribute to the soup's full and nutritional quality.

• **Fresh veggies**: Use a variety of fresh veggies such as carrots, celery, spinach, zucchini and tomatoes. These provide flavour, texture, and vitamins.

• Whole Grains: For more fibre and energy, try quinoa, brown rice, or barley.

• **Herbs and Spices**: Add flavour with fresh herbs and spices such as parsley, cilantro, thyme, rosemary, garlic, and ginger. These not only enhance flavour but also provide health benefits.

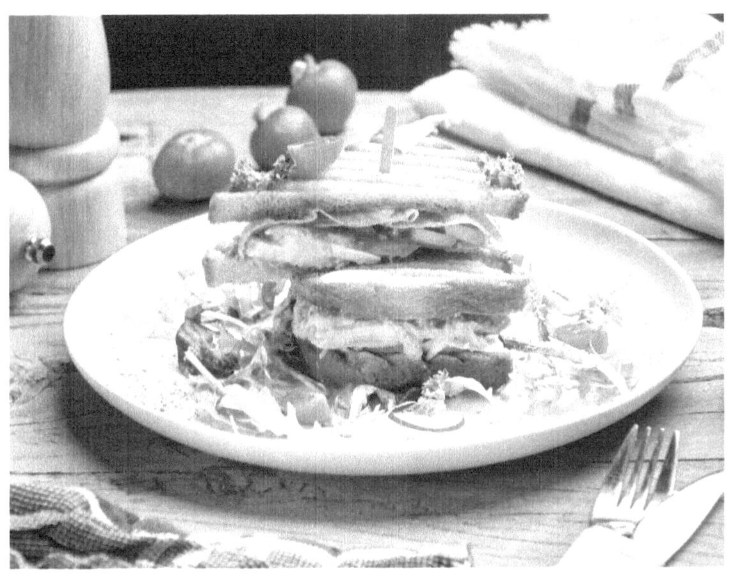

Wholesome Sandwiches and Wraps

Sandwiches and wraps can be quick, convenient, and nutritious lunch options if prepared properly.

• Wholegrain Bread: Select whole-grain bread, wraps, or pita pockets. These selections contain more fibre and minerals than refined white bread.

• **Fresh Vegetables:** Stock up on lettuce, spinach, tomatoes, cucumbers, bell peppers, and sprouts. These provide crunch and nutrition.

• **Flavour enhancers**: Use mustard, hummus, pesto, or a little vinaigrette. Avoid sugary sauces and condiments.

• **Portion Control:** If you're creating a large sandwich or wrap, try halving it and keeping the rest for later or sharing it. This helps to control portion sizes.

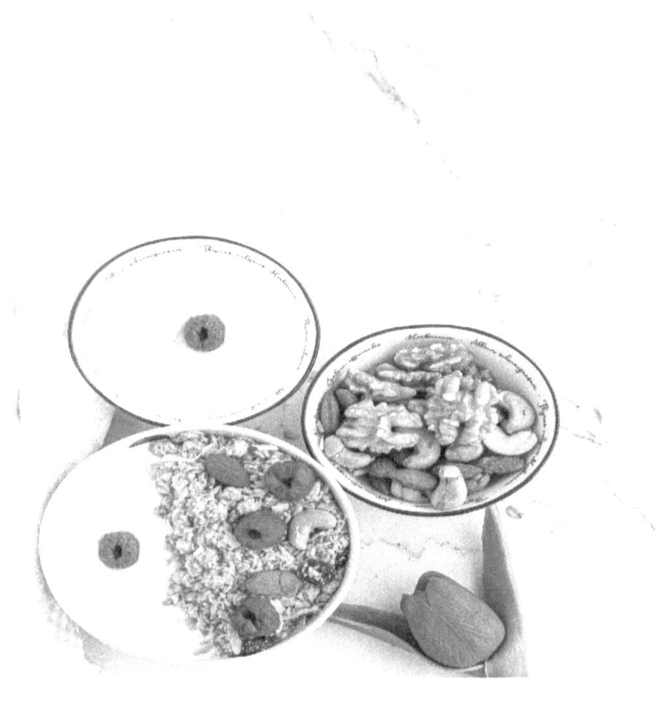

Grain Bowls and Power Plates

Grain bowls and power plates are adaptable and nutrient-dense, combining multiple food categories to provide a well-balanced meal.

• **Whole Grain Base**: Begin with whole grains such as quinoa, brown rice, farro, or barley. These grains contain complex carbs and fibre, which provide long-term energy.

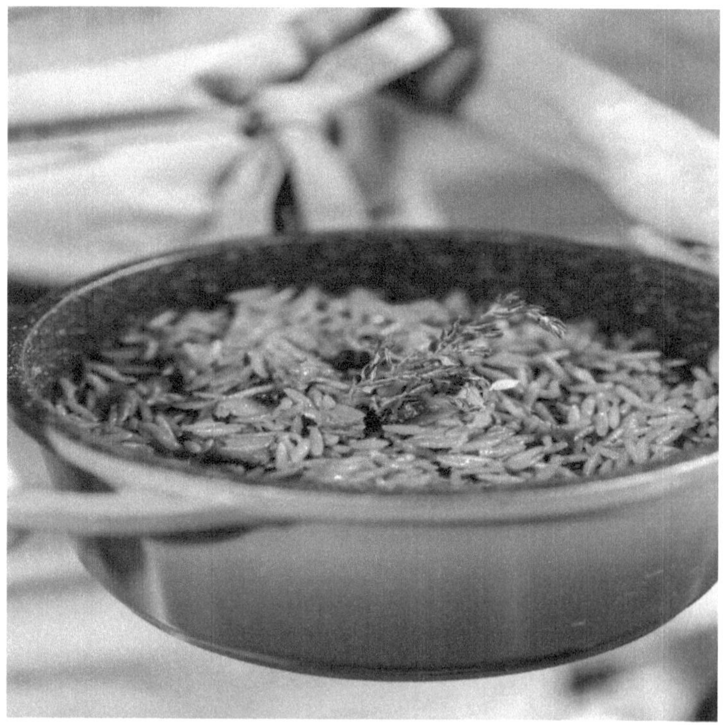

• **Colourful veggies:** Use a mix of raw and cooked veggies, such as roasted sweet potatoes, steamed broccoli, shredded carrots, and sautéed spinach. This enhances flavour, texture, and nutrition.

• **Garnishes:** Use fresh herbs, a squeeze of lemon juice, or a sprinkling of feta cheese. These final touches improve the overall flavour character.

Incorporate robust salads and soups, nourishing sandwiches and wraps, and nutrient-rich grain bowls and power plates into your lunch routine for tasty and balanced meals that support your health and keep you energised throughout the day.

11. Nourishing dinners

Protein-Rich Main Courses

Protein is required to maintain muscle mass, promote metabolism, and keep you pleased. Here are some suggestions for protein-rich dinners:

• **Grilled Chicken Breast:** Marinate chicken breasts with olive oil, lemon juice, garlic, and spices. Grill till juicy and tender. Serve with steamed vegetables and quinoa for a well-balanced lunch.

• **Baked Salmon:** Sprinkle salmon fillets with salt, pepper, and a squeeze of lemon. Bake till flaky, then serve with a fresh salad and roasted sweet potatoes. Salmon contains omega-3 fatty acids, which are helpful to heart health.

• **Turkey Meatballs:** Mix ground turkey, minced onions, garlic, breadcrumbs, and egg. Roll into balls and bake. Serve with tomato-based sauce and whole grain pasta. This recipe is lower in fat than typical beef meatballs.

• **Shrimp Stir-Fry**: Cook shrimp with bell peppers, snap peas, and broccoli in a garlic-soy sauce. Serve with brown rice. This recipe is quick, flavourful, and full of lean protein.

• **Beef and Vegetable** Skewers: Thread lean beef cubes, cherry tomatoes, bell peppers, and onions on skewers. Grill the steak until it is cooked to your preference. Serve with a side of couscous.

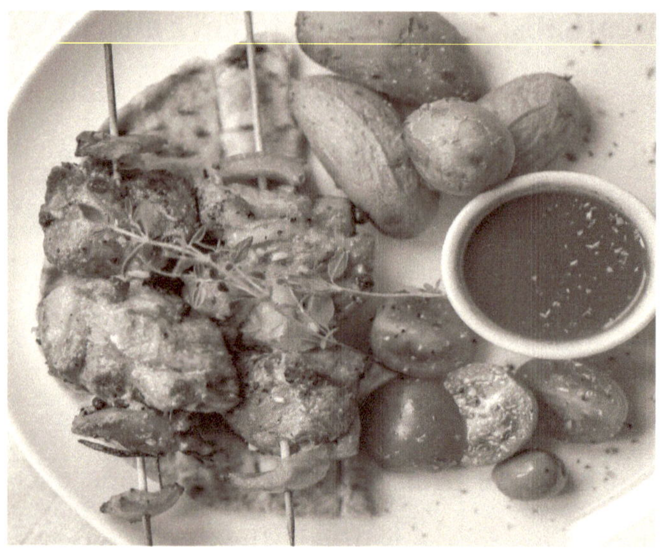

Flavourful Vegetarian Options

Flavourful Vegetarian Options

Vegetarian meals can be both fulfilling and nourishing. Here are some flavourful and nutritious meal ideas:

• **Vegetable Stir-Fry:** Sauté a mixture of your favourite veggies, such as bell peppers, broccoli, carrots, and snap peas, in a soy ginger sauce. Serve with brown rice or quinoa. For more protein, add tofu.

• **Chickpea and Spinach Curry:** Cook chickpeas in a rich tomato sauce with spinach, onions, garlic, and a spice blend including cumin, coriander, and turmeric. Serve alongside basmati rice or whole wheat naan.

• **Stuffed Bell Peppers:** Combine quinoa, black beans, corn, chopped tomatoes, and spices. Bake the peppers until they're soft. If wanted, put some cheese on top.

• **Lentil Shepherd's Pie**: Combine cooked lentils, carrots, peas and corn in a savoury gravy. Top with mashed cauliflower or potatoes and bake till golden. This dish is hearty and comforting.

• **Mushroom and Spinach Risotto:** Prepare arborio rice by sautéing mushrooms, spinach, onions, garlic, and vegetable broth. To add richness, stir in a little Parmesan cheese. This risotto is rich and satisfying.

Enjoy comfort meals with a healthy spin. These makeovers preserve the flavours you enjoy while providing higher nutrition:

• **Cauliflower Crust Pizza:** Instead of using regular dough, make a cauliflower crust. Top with marinara sauce, mozzarella, and your preferred vegetables. Bake until the cheese is melted and bubbly.

• **Zucchini Noodles with Marinara:** Instead of pasta, use spiralized zucchini noodles. Toss in homemade marinara sauce and turkey meatballs.

This recipe is minimal in carbohydrates but strong in flavour.

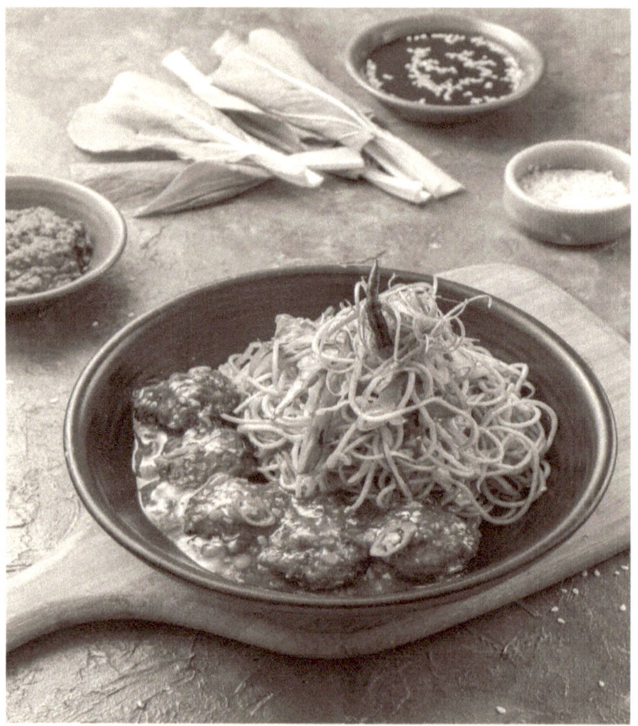

• **Baked Sweet Potato Fries:** Cut sweet potatoes into wedges, drizzle with olive oil, salt, and pepper, then bake until crispy. Present with a side of Greek yoghurt dip. These fries are a healthier alternative to the standard fries.

• **Quinoa Mac and Cheese:** Instead of pasta, make a lighter cheese sauce with Greek yoghurt and a touch of cheddar. This dish is heavy in protein but low in carbohydrates.

• **Turkey Chilli:** Make chilli with ground turkey, beans, tomatoes, and a spice mix. Serve with a serving of whole grain cornbread. This version contains less fat while remaining substantial and filling.

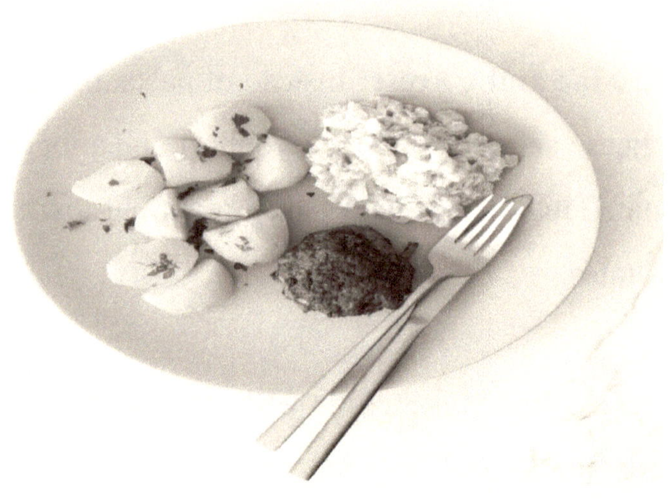

Incorporate protein-packed main courses, flavourful vegetarian options, and comfort food makeovers into your evening routine to enjoy tasty and healthy meals that promote your health and well-being.

12. Healthy Snacks and Treats.

Nutritional Snack Ideas

Snacking wisely is critical for keeping energy levels stable and avoiding overeating at meals. Here are some healthy and delicious snack options:

• **Fresh Fruit with Nut Butter:** Pairing apple slices, bananas, or celery sticks with almond or peanut butter creates a pleasant and filling snack. The fruit gives natural sugars and fibre, while the nut butter contains protein and healthy fats.

• **Greek Yoghurt with Berries:** A bowl of Greek yoghurt topped with fresh berries is an excellent source of protein, antioxidants, and vitamins. To add extra crunch, sprinkle with nuts or seeds.

- **Hummus and Veggies:** Cut up colourful veggies such as carrots, bell peppers, cucumbers, and cherry tomatoes. Dip them in hummus for a fiber-rich snack with plant-based protein.

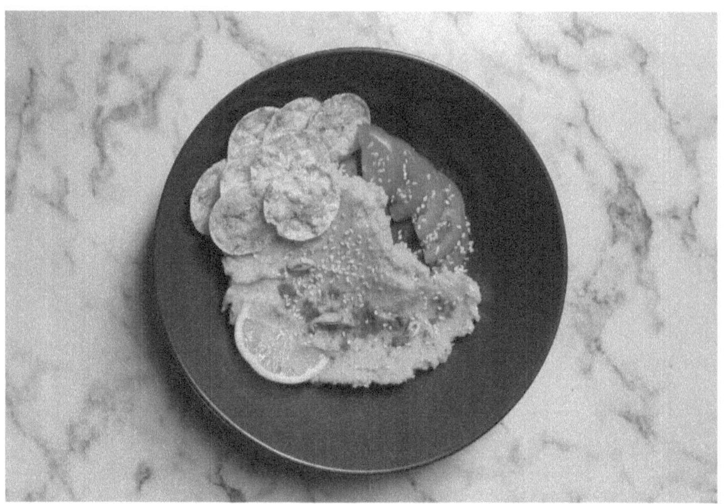

- **Whole Grain Crackers and Cheese:** Choose whole grain crackers and pair them with a slice of cheese for a snack that mixes complex carbohydrates with protein. This mixture is both satisfying and delicious.

• **Hard-Boiled Eggs:** Store a few hard-boiled eggs in the refrigerator for a quick and protein-rich snack. Sprinkle with salt and pepper, or serve with a dollop of mustard.

A sweet treat does not have to disrupt your healthy eating habits. Here are some great dessert recipes that you may enjoy guilt-free:

• **Chia Pudding:** Combine chia seeds, almond milk, and a little of honey. Allow it to sit in the refrigerator overnight until it thickens into a custard. Finish with fresh berries or a sprinkling of cinnamon.

• **Dark Chocolate:** Select chocolate with at least 70% cocoa content. A tiny slice can satisfy your sweet taste while also containing antioxidants and flavonoids.

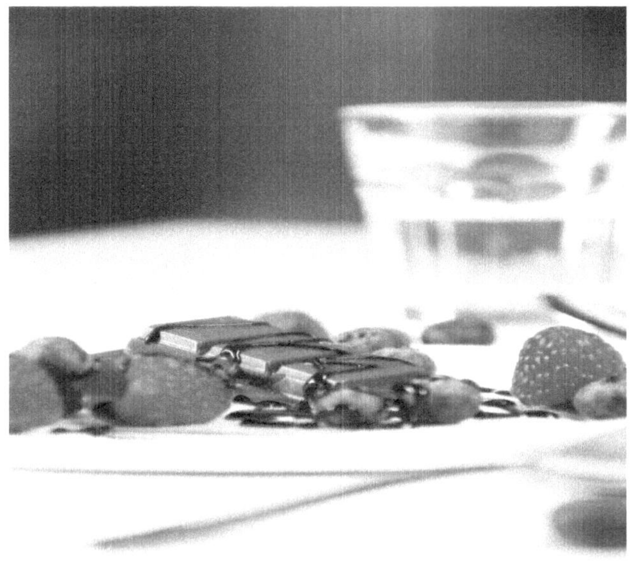

• **Frozen Yoghurt Bark:** Spread Greek yoghurt on a baking sheet, then top with nuts, seeds, and berries. Freeze until solid. Tear into pieces for a refreshing and crispy delight.

• **Baked Apples:** Core one apple and fill with oats, cinnamon, and a drizzle of honey. Bake the apples until they are soft and the filling is golden.

- **Avocado Chocolate Mousse:** Combine ripe avocado, chocolate powder, a drizzle of honey or maple syrup, and a splash of vanilla extract. This creamy treat is high in beneficial fats and antioxidants.

Smart Options for Cravings

Managing cravings is essential for keeping a healthy diet. Here are some good options to help you keep on track:

• **Craving Crunch:** Replace potato chips with air-popped popcorn. Season with nutritional yeast, garlic powder, or a sprinkling of Parmesan cheese for a savoury, low-calorie snack high in fibre.

• **Sweet cravings? Satisfy** them with a piece of fruit or a handful of berries. These natural sweets are rich in vitamins, minerals, and fibre and have no added sugars.

• **Have a salty craving?** Try roasted chickpeas instead of pretzels or salted nuts. Season with spices such as paprika or cumin for a crispy, protein-rich snack.

• **Craving something creamy**? Blend Greek yoghurt, spinach, a frozen banana, and a splash of almond milk. This creamy beverage is loaded with protein, fibre, and minerals.

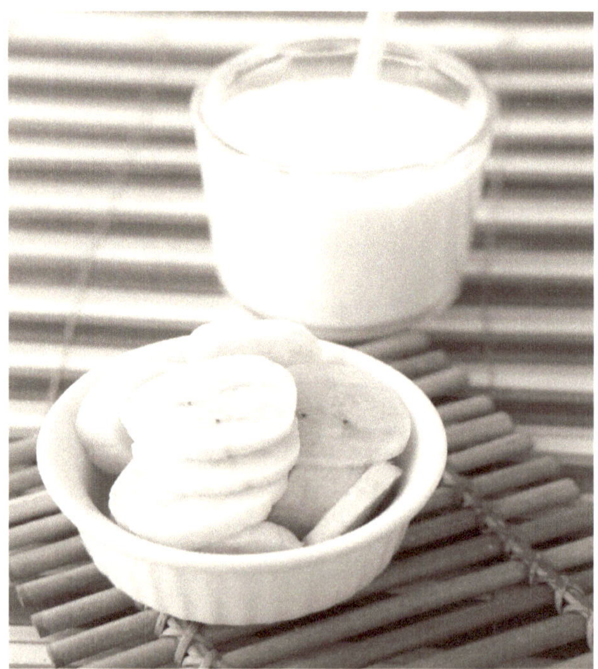

• **Craving chocolate?** Try a small portion of dark chocolate or a handmade hot cocoa made with unsweetened cocoa powder, almond milk, and a touch of honey.

You may enjoy delicious foods while also supporting your health and wellness objectives if you incorporate these healthy snack options, guilt-free treats, and smart cravings choices into your daily routine.

Part V: Lifestyle and Long-Term Success: Integrating Physical Activity

13. Benefits of Exercise for Diabetes

Regular physical activity is essential for treating diabetes efficiently. Exercise provides several benefits, including:

• **Improved Blood Sugar Control:** Physical exercise helps your muscles use glucose for energy, which lowers blood sugar levels. This can enhance glycaemic management and lower the risk of diabetic complications.

• **Increased Insulin Sensitivity:** Exercise makes your body's cells more receptive to insulin, reducing the amount of insulin required to control blood sugar levels.

• **Weight Management:** Regular activity burns calories, which is necessary for weight loss or maintaining a healthy weight. This is especially essential for those with type 2 diabetes because weight management is closely related to better blood sugar control.

• **Cardiovascular Health:** Physical activity strengthens the heart and improves circulation, lowering the risk of heart disease, a significant side effect of diabetes.

• **Mental Health:** Exercise produces endorphins, which can improve mood while reducing stress and anxiety. This mental health advantage is critical for overall wellness and diabetes management.

• **Increased Energy Levels:** Regular exercise increases energy and lowers exhaustion, making it simpler to stay active throughout the day.

Physical Activities to Consider

When incorporating exercise into your daily schedule, make sure to choose things you enjoy. Here are some examples of physical activities to consider:

• **Aerobic Exercise:** Walking, jogging, cycling, and swimming raise your heart rate and promote cardiovascular health. Aim to complete at least 150 minutes of moderate-intensity aerobic activity every week.

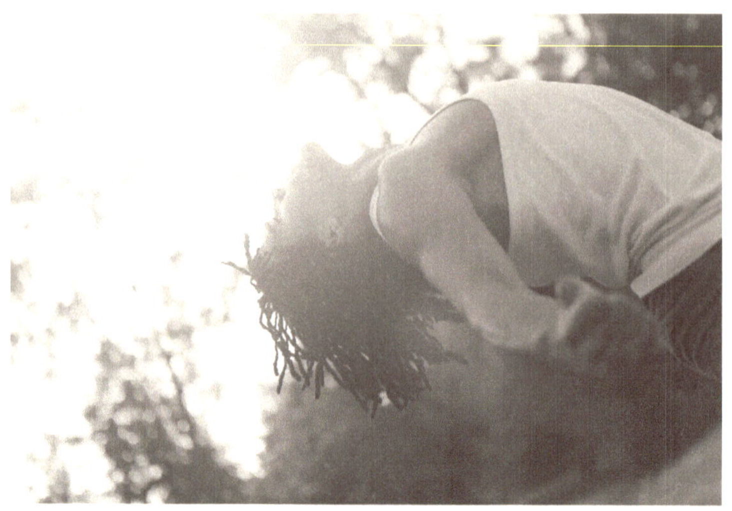

• **Strength Training:** Lifting weights or utilising resistance bands increases muscular mass and strength. This form of exercise also helps to maintain healthy bones and joints.

• **Flexibility exercises:** Yoga and stretching can help you increase your flexibility and range of motion. These exercises can help to avoid injuries and improve general physical function.

• **Balance Exercises:** Practicing balance exercises, such as tai chi or balance-focused yoga positions, can help prevent falls and improve coordination.

• **High-Intensity Interval Training (HIIT):** HIIT consists of short bursts of intense activity followed by rest or low-intensity exercise. This sort of exercise can be quite successful at increasing fitness and burning calories in a shorter period of time.

Creating an Exercise Routine.

Creating a consistent exercise regimen will help you stay on track towards your health objectives. Here's how to set up an efficient routine:

- **Set realistic goals.** Begin with realistic goals depending on your current fitness level. Gradually increase the intensity and duration of your workouts as you gain comfort and fitness.

- **Plan Regular Workouts:** Treat your workout sessions like any other important appointment. Aim for 30 minutes of physical activity most days of the week.

- **Change Up Your Activities:** Include a variety of exercises to keep your program interesting and engage different muscle groups. This variety might help you avoid boredom and stay motivated.

• **Listen to Your Body:** Pay attention to how your body reacts to exercise. If you experience pain or extreme weariness, take a rest or change your activity to avoid harm.

• **Stay Hydrated and Eat Well:** Proper hydration and nutrition are critical for fuelling workouts and promoting recovery. Drink plenty of water and consume balanced meals with carbohydrates, proteins, and healthy fats.

• **Track Your Progress:** Keep a track of your workouts and progress. This might help you stay motivated and track your progress.

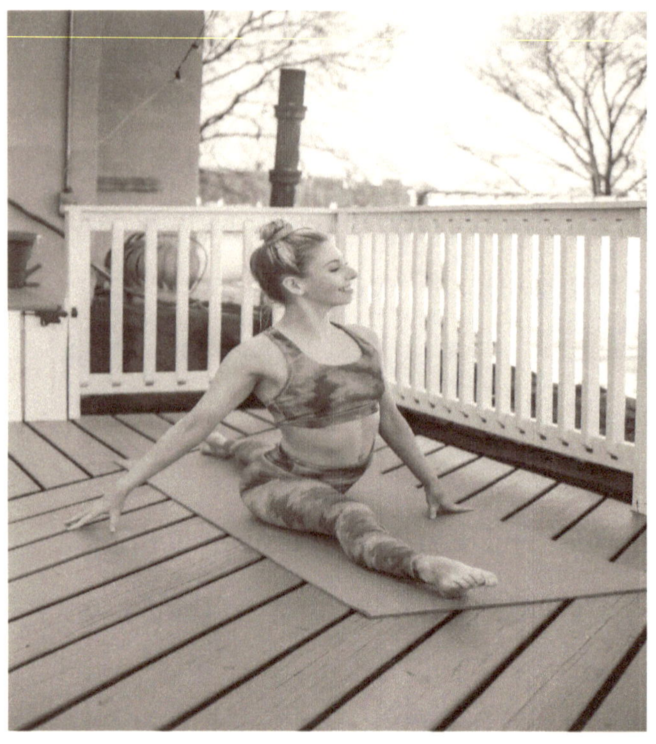

Regular physical activity can help manage diabetes and enhance overall health. Understanding the benefits, trying out different sorts of workouts, and developing a well-rounded regimen will help you achieve long-term success and a healthy future.

14. Managing Stress and Emotional Wellbeing

The Relationship Between Stress and Blood Sugar

Stress can have a major impact on blood sugar levels, especially among diabetics. When the body is stressed, it produces stress hormones such as cortisol and adrenaline.

These hormones prime the body for a "fight or flight" reaction, causing the liver to pump more glucose into the bloodstream for immediate energy. For diabetics, this can result in increased blood sugar.

Additionally, stress might influence behaviours that affect diabetes treatment. When people are worried, they may skip meals, overeat, or reach for harmful comfort foods. Sleep habits might also be interrupted, complicating blood glucose regulation. Understanding the relationship between stress and blood sugar is critical for successful diabetes treatment.

Meditation and Relaxation Techniques

Mindfulness and relaxation exercises can help relieve stress and promote emotional well-being. These activities can improve blood sugar control by reducing stress hormone levels and instilling a sense of calm.

• **Mindful Breathing:** Deep, slow breaths might assist to relax the nervous system and relieve tension. Concentrate on your breathing, inhale deeply through your nose and exhale gently through your mouth. Practise for a few minutes each day.

• **Meditation:** Engaging in regular meditation can help reduce stress and enhance mental clarity. Locate a peaceful location to sit comfortably, close your eyes, and concentrate on your breath or mantra. Begin with a few minutes every day and progressively increase the duration.

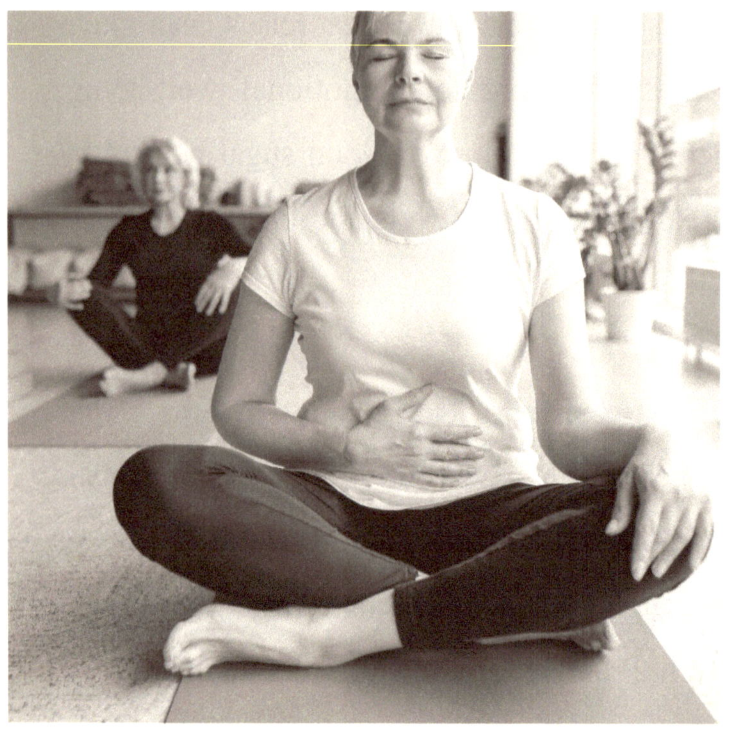

• **Progressive Muscle Relaxation:**

This technique involves tensing and then gradually relaxing various muscle groups throughout the body. Begin with your toes and work your way up to your head, focussing on relieving tension in each place.

• **Yoga:** Yoga combines physical postures, breathing exercises, and meditation to alleviate stress while increasing flexibility and strength. Regular practice can help reduce stress hormone levels and enhance feelings of well-being.

• **Guided Imagery:** Imagine a relaxing and pleasant setting, such as a beach or forest. Close your eyes and visualise yourself in this environment, concentrating on the sights, sounds, and scents. This technique can help to alleviate stress and promote relaxation.

Building a Support System

Having a solid support system is essential for managing diabetes and staying emotionally well. Support can be provided by family, friends, healthcare professionals, and community services. Here's how to create and maintain a support system:

• **Family & Friends:** Communicate your diabetes control goals to your loved ones. Their understanding and encouragement can be really beneficial. Don't be afraid to ask for help when you need it, whether it's emotional support or practical assistance.

• **Support Groups:** Participating in a diabetes support group, whether in person or online, can help you feel more connected and share your experiences. Connecting with individuals who understand your situation can provide support and advice.

- **Healthcare Team:** Regular communication with your healthcare providers is essential. They can provide advice, track your progress, and help you change your treatment plan as necessary. Please do not hesitate to contact them if you have any queries or issues.

- **Community Resources:** Locate local or online resources that include educational workshops, fitness classes, or dietary counselling. These resources can offer additional assistance and information to help you manage your diabetes properly.

- **Mental Health Professionals:** If stress or emotional difficulties become unbearable, get assistance from a therapist or counsellor. They may teach you coping methods for stress, anxiety, and depression, as well as help you establish a healthy mentality.

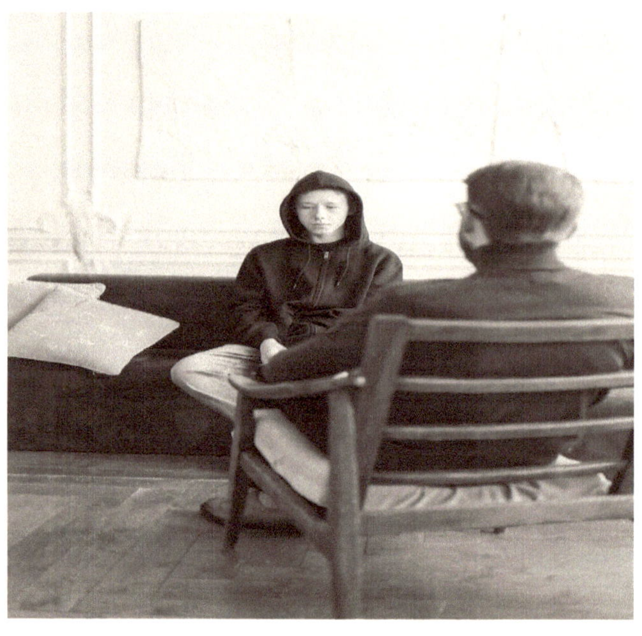

Understanding the relationship between stress and blood sugar, practicing mindfulness and relaxation techniques, and developing a strong support system can help you manage diabetes and enhance your overall emotional well-being. Taking these actions can result in a better, more balanced lifestyle.

15. Monitor Your Progress

Monitor Blood Sugar Levels

Monitoring blood sugar levels is an important element of managing diabetes. Regular tracking helps you understand how various foods, activities, and medications affect your glucose levels, allowing you to make more informed health decisions.

• **Using a Glucometer:** A glucometer is a device that measures blood sugar levels from a little drop of blood, usually obtained through a finger prick. To get reliable readings, follow the instructions that came with your glucometer. Keep a continuous record of your blood sugar readings, noting the time of day and any related events, such as meals or exercise.

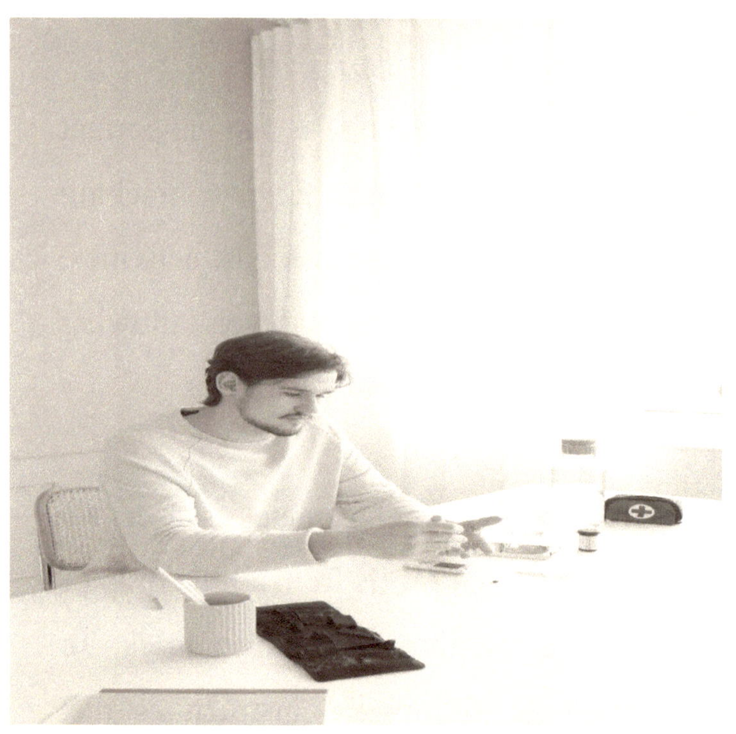

• **Continuous Glucose Monitors (CGMs):** CGMs are wearable devices that measure blood sugar levels in real time throughout the day and night. They are made up of a sensor embedded under the skin that sends data to a monitor or smartphone. CGMs can provide a comprehensive view of your glucose patterns and trends, allowing you to identify fluctuations and adapt your management strategy accordingly.

• **Keeping a journal:** Keeping a journal or utilising a digital app to track your blood sugar levels, as well as other factors like food intake, physical activity, stress, and medication, might provide useful information. Regularly reviewing this data with your healthcare team can help you find patterns and areas for improvement.

Understanding Your Laboratory Results

Regular lab testing are an important aspect of controlling diabetes. These tests provide precise information about your overall health and how well your diabetes is managed.

• **Haemoglobin A1c (HbA1c):** This test measures your average blood sugar levels throughout the previous two to three months.. It provides a long-term perspective on your glucose control. Most people with diabetes aim for a HbA1c level of 7% or lower, however your healthcare practitioner may recommend a different goal based on your specific needs.

• **Fasting Blood Glucose:** This test determines your blood sugar levels after an overnight fast. It helps determine how well your body regulates glucose in the absence of recent meals. A fasting blood glucose level of less than 100 mg/dL is considered normal; levels between 100 and 125 mg/dL suggest prediabetes, while levels of 126 mg/dL or more indicate diabetes.

• **Lipid Profile:** This test measures cholesterol and triglyceride levels. People with diabetes are more likely to develop heart disease, so it is critical to monitor their cardiovascular health. The lipid profile consists of total cholesterol, LDL (bad) cholesterol, HDL (good) cholesterol, and triglycerides. Maintaining healthy levels can help lower your chance of problems.

• **Kidney Function Tests:** The urine albumin-to-creatinine ratio (UACR) and serum creatinine levels assess kidney function. Diabetes can harm the kidneys, thus tracking these levels might help detect early signs of kidney impairment.

Adjusting Your Plan for Continued Success

Diabetes management is a continuous process that necessitates frequent modifications to ensure optimal health. Here's how to maintain your strategy effective and adaptable:

• **Schedule regular check-ins with your healthcare team**. Make regular consultations with your doctor to discuss your blood sugar levels, lab findings, and overall health. These check-ins allow you to make any necessary changes to your treatment plan, such as changes in medication, food, or physical exercise.

• **Creating and Revising Goals:** Set precise, attainable objectives for your diabetes management. These could include goals for blood sugar control, weight loss, or physical activity. Review and alter these goals as appropriate based on your success and new health information.

- **Staying Informed:** Diabetes research and treatment options are constantly evolving. Attending educational programs, joining support groups, or reading credible sources might help you stay up to date on new developments. Knowledge enables you to make informed decisions regarding your health.

- **Adapting to Life Changes:** Major life events, such as changes in job, travel, or family dynamics, can all have an impact on diabetes management. Be prepared to change your routine to accommodate new situations. Flexibility and early planning can help to keep blood sugar levels consistent during transitions.

- **Listening to Your Body:** Notice how your body reacts to various foods, activities, and stressors. If you detect any patterns or changes, speak with your healthcare professional. Your body can provide useful input as you refine your management strategy.

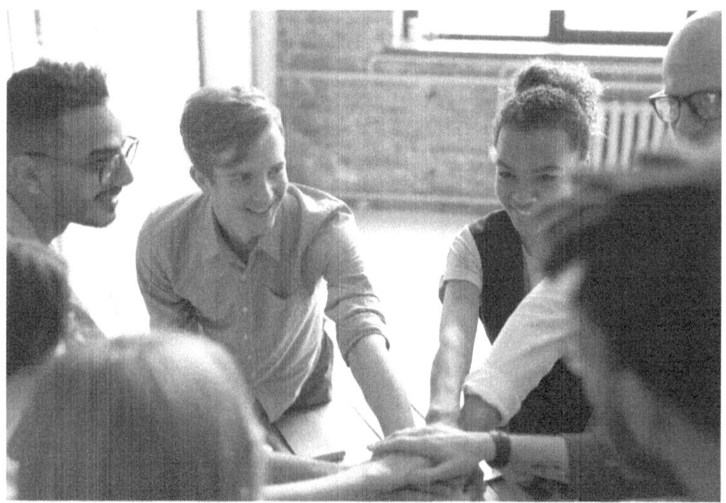

You can achieve long-term success in diabetes control by diligently measuring blood sugar levels, evaluating test results, and adjusting your management strategy as needed. This proactive approach promotes general well-being and prevents difficulties, resulting in a healthier and more balanced lifestyle.

Conclusion/ *Bonus*

Your Journey to Reversal and Beyond

Keeping Yourself Motivated and Inspired To overcome diabetes and continue living a healthy lifestyle requires a significant commitment at the outset. It is essential for long-term success to maintain inspiration and motivation.

Keep in mind why you started this journey: for your future, your loved ones, and health. Be surrounded by positive people, whether they are supportive family members, friends, or a group of people who are working toward the same goals. Celebrate small wins en route to see the value in your advancement. Take into consideration the positive changes in your mood, energy, and overall well-being. During trying times, these reflections can assist you in regaining your motivation.

Tips for Long-Term Maintenance Keeping your progress going requires a consistent, balanced approach. The following are some useful strategies for long-term success:

• **Continuity is essential:** Keep to your healthy eating, exercise, and monitoring schedule. Habits are formed through consistency, making it simpler to maintain progress without becoming overwhelmed.

• **Stay Up to Date:** Continue to find out about diabetes the executives, sustenance, and new exploration. With this information, you can adapt to changes in your condition or way of life with confidence.

• **Adaptability and transformation:** Life is full of changes and unexpected events. Be ready to adjust your routine to accommodate new circumstances, like a tight work schedule, travel, or social events. Flexibility helps you stay on course and avoid additional stress.

• **Regular Examinations:** Keep in touch with your doctor on a regular basis to keep track of your progress, make changes to your treatment plan, and deal with problems. Interventions can be carried out quickly when potential issues are identified early.

• **Careful Eating:** Take note of your body's signals of fullness and hunger. Mindful eating prevents overeating and fosters a positive relationship with food.

• **Active work:** Remain moving! In addition to lowering blood sugar levels, regular exercise boosts mood and overall health. Make fitness a joyful and necessary part of your life by engaging in activities you enjoy.

• **Stress the board:** Engage in stress-reduction activities like yoga, mindfulness, and meditation. Your overall health and blood sugar levels benefit from stress management.

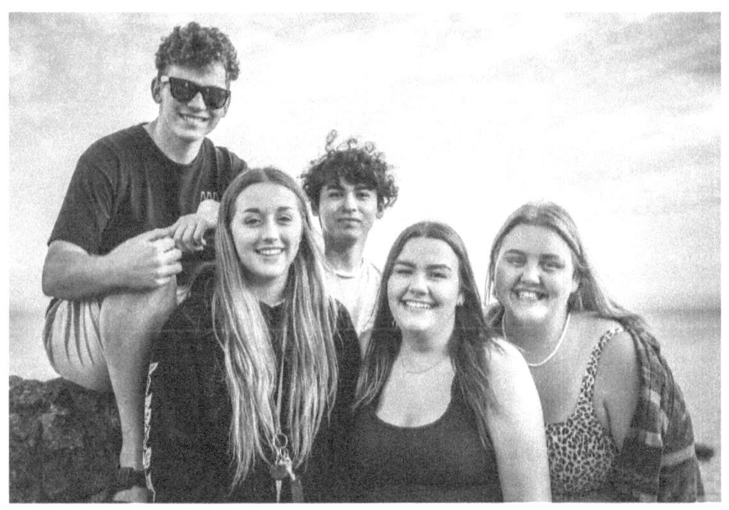

Celebrating your achievements in health.

Praising your wellbeing achievements is a pivotal part of staying roused and valuing your diligent effort. Even if they seem insignificant, take the time to notice and celebrate your accomplishments. The following are a few techniques to respect your achievements:

• **Consider your journey:** Think about where you began and how far you've come. You might find that reflecting on your trip made you feel successful and motivated to continue.

• **Set objectives:** Break down your long-term objectives into more manageable steps. Praise every achievement with something interesting, like a treat, another activity gadget, or a three day weekend to depressurize and recuperate.

• **Share your achievement:** Communicate your progress to family, friends, and support groups. Praising with others builds your mentality, yet it might assist with spurring others around you.

• **Treat Yourself Well:** Give yourself non-food rewards that make you happy, like a new book, a spa day, or an activity you've wanted to do for a long time.

• **Keep Track of Your Progress:** Keep a scrapbook or journal of your journey with pictures, notes, and successes. This genuine record could act as a wake up call of your work and commitment.

Final Thoughts

Switching diabetes and laying out a solid way of life requests responsibility, tolerance, and industriousness. It is possible to achieve long-term health and well-being by being driven, adjusting to changes, and taking pleasure in your accomplishments.

Keep in mind that this involves more than just treating a disease; It's about being happier and healthier. Keep yourself informed, celebrate each step, and never underestimate the power of your dedication and effort. Your excursion to diabetes inversion is more than simply an objective; it is a lifetime obligation to your wellbeing and future.

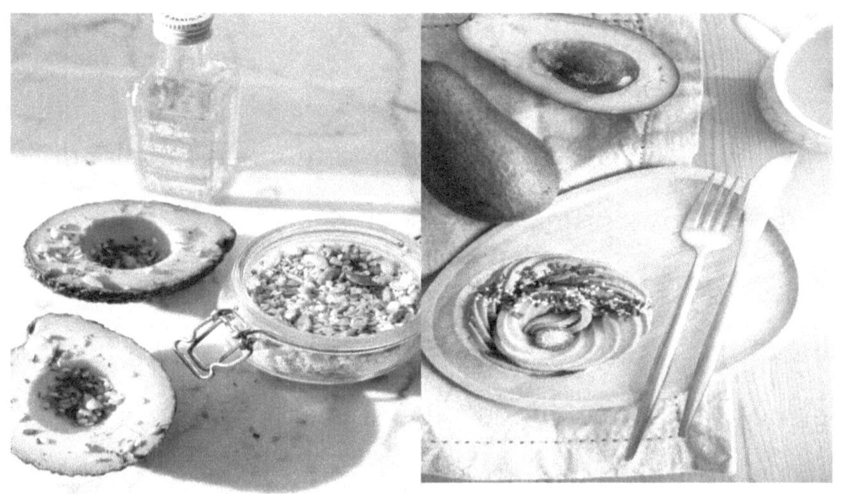

Appendices

Glossary of Key Terms

• **A1C (Hemoglobin A1c):** A blood test that measures your average blood sugar levels over the past 2-3 months. It's used to diagnose and monitor diabetes.

• **Blood Glucose:** The main sugar found in the blood and the body's primary source of energy.

• **Carbohydrates:** Nutrients found in foods like bread, pasta, and fruits, which are broken down into glucose and affect blood sugar levels.

• **Continuous Glucose Monitor (CGM):** A device that tracks glucose levels in real-time throughout the day and night.

• **Diabetes Mellitus:** A group of diseases that result in high blood sugar due to the body's inability to produce or use insulin effectively.

• **Fasting Blood Glucose:** A test that measures blood sugar levels after not eating or drinking (except water) for at least 8 hours.

• **Gestational Diabetes:** A form of diabetes that occurs during pregnancy and usually goes away after the baby is born.

• **Hyperglycemia:** Higher than normal blood sugar levels.

• **Hypoglycemia:** Lower than normal blood sugar levels.

• **Insulin:** A hormone produced by the pancreas that helps glucose enter cells for energy.

• **Type 1 Diabetes:** An autoimmune condition where the body attacks insulin-producing cells in the pancreas, leading to little or no insulin production.

• **Type 2 Diabetes:** A condition where the body becomes resistant to insulin or doesn't produce enough insulin, often linked to lifestyle factors.

Additional Resources and Reading

• **Books:**

• "Dr. Bernstein's Diabetes Solution" by Dr. Richard K. Bernstein

• "The End of Diabetes" by Dr. Joel Fuhrman

• "The Diabetes Code" by Dr. Jason Fung

• **Websites:**

• American Diabetes Association: www.diabetes.org

• Mayo Clinic - Diabetes Management: www.mayoclinic.org

• Diabetes UK: www.diabetes.org.uk

• **Support Groups:**

• Diabetes Daily Forum: www.diabetesdaily.com/forum

• JDRF (Juvenile Diabetes Research Foundation): www.jdrf.org

• **Apps:**

• **MySugr:** A diabetes logbook app for tracking blood sugar, carbs, and more.

• **Glucose Buddy:** An app for tracking blood sugar levels, medications, and meals.

• **Carb Manager**: A comprehensive app for tracking carbs and managing a diabetes-friendly diet.

References

Bernstein, R. K. (2011). Dr. Bernstein's Diabetes Solution: The Complete Guide to Achieving Normal Blood Sugars. Little, Brown Spark.

Fung, J. (2018). The Diabetes Code: Prevent and Reverse Type 2 Diabetes Naturally. Greystone Books.

Fuhrman, J. (2012). The End of Diabetes: The Eat to Live Plan to Prevent and Reverse Diabetes. HarperOne.